THE CORTISOL DETOX DIET PLAN

Reset Your Hormones, Boost Energy, and Lose Weight Naturally with Proven Strategies and 21-Day Meal Plans for Optimal Health

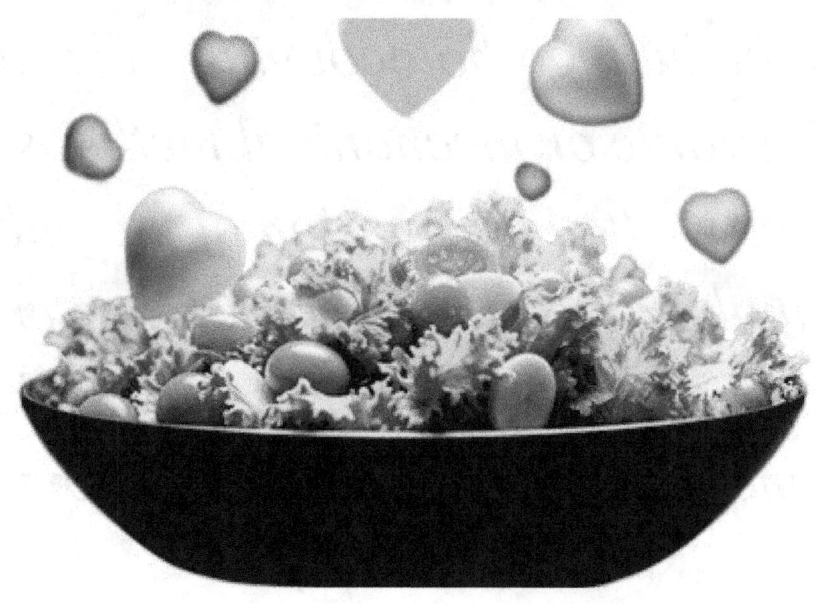

SALLY S. KELLEY

TABLE OF CONTENTS

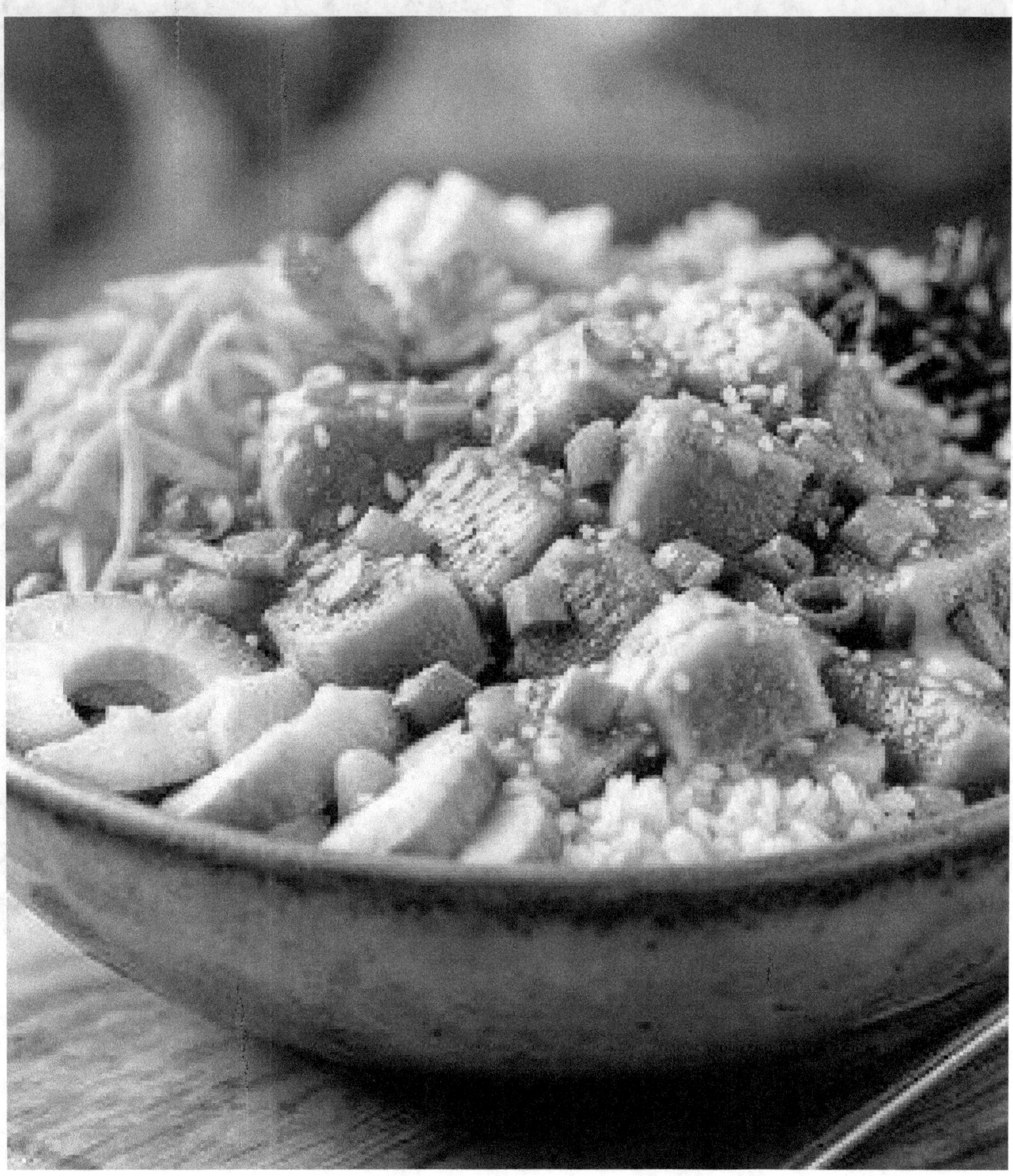

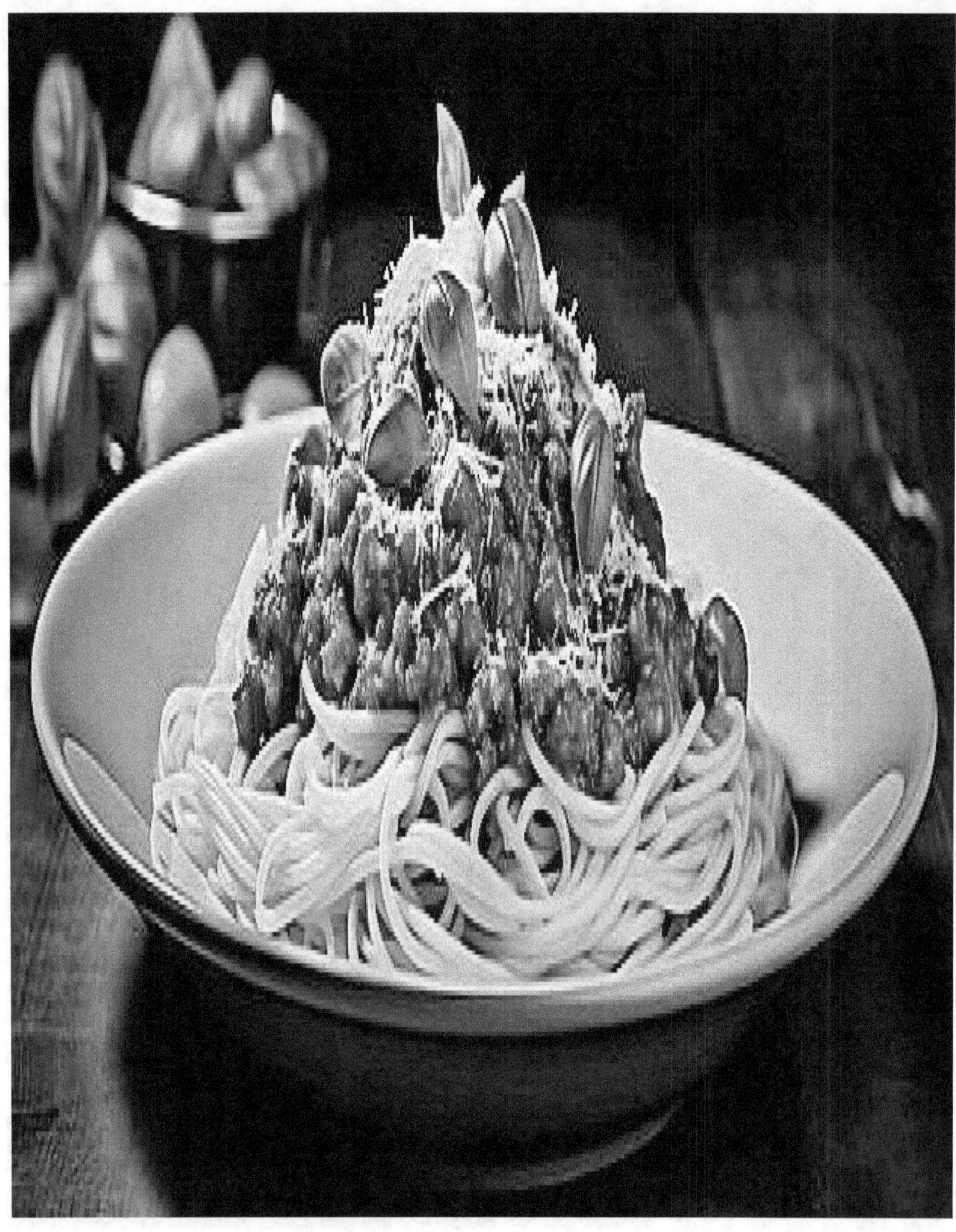

INTRODUCTION

In today's fast-paced world, stress has become a constant part of our lives. Whether it's work pressures, family responsibilities, or just the demands of daily living, stress can take a serious toll on our health. One of the most affected areas is our hormones, and at the center of this is a hormone called cortisol.

Cortisol is often referred to as the "stress hormone" because it's released when we feel stressed. While cortisol is important for regulating our body's response to stress, when it's constantly elevated due to long-term stress, it can cause several problems. High cortisol levels can lead to weight gain, poor sleep, mood swings, and even weaken the immune system. Over time, this imbalance can increase your risk for more serious health issues, such as heart disease, diabetes, and chronic fatigue.

The Cortisol Detox Diet Plan is designed to help you reset your body and lower those stress hormones. This plan focuses on foods and habits that support your adrenal glands (the organs responsible for producing cortisol), reduce inflammation, and bring balance to your hormone levels. It includes nutrient-rich meals that are not only good for your body but also help you feel calmer and more energized.

By following this plan, you can begin to take control of your health and feel better both physically and emotionally. You'll notice improved sleep, more stable moods, and better weight management. The goal is not just to lower cortisol but to create lasting habits that will help you feel balanced and healthy long term. This isn't about dieting—it's about adopting a lifestyle that nurtures your body and mind, helping you handle stress with more ease and living your life with greater vitality.

Let's dive into the Cortisol Detox Diet Plan and explore how making small, positive changes can bring big results for your health.

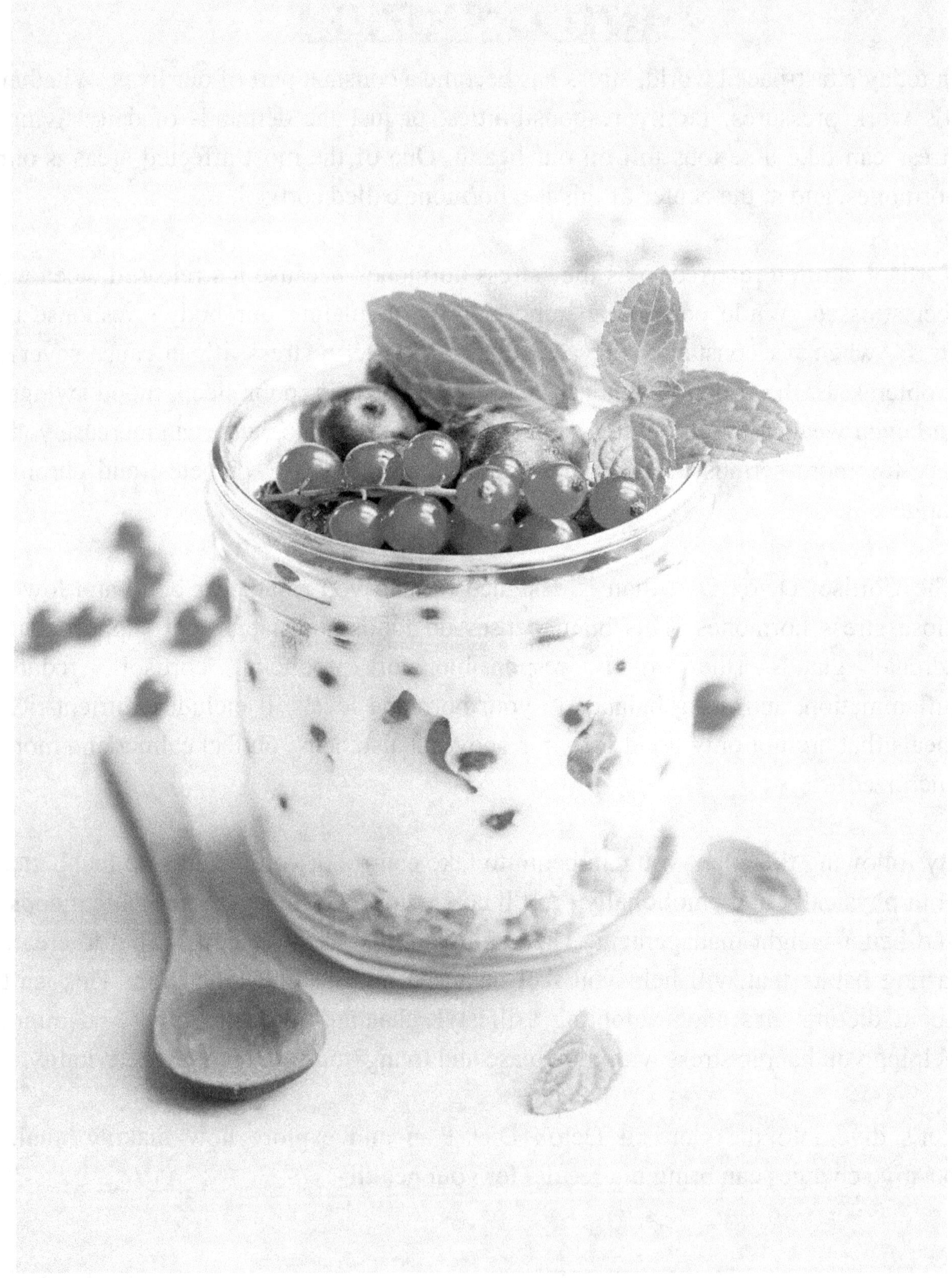

CHAPTER 1

What Is Cortisol and Why It Matters

Cortisol is one of the most important hormones in your body, often referred to as the "stress hormone." It plays a vital role in a wide range of bodily functions, including regulating metabolism, the immune response, and blood pressure. Produced by the adrenal glands, cortisol is essential for your survival, helping your body respond to stress, maintain energy levels, and perform well under pressure. However, its impact goes far beyond merely managing stress—it's a fundamental regulator of health.

When your body perceives a stressor—whether physical, emotional, or environmental—cortisol is released to help you react quickly. In the short term, this stress response is helpful and necessary. Cortisol increases the release of glucose into the bloodstream, providing your muscles and brain with the energy they need to fight or flee. It also helps you focus, heightens alertness, and reduces pain sensitivity.

However, while cortisol has a vital protective role, the issue arises when cortisol levels remain elevated for extended periods due to chronic stress. That's when cortisol becomes more of a problem than a solution.

Cortisol and Its Impact on Health

When cortisol levels are chronically high, they can wreak havoc on your body and mind. Here's how this hormone can negatively affect different aspects of health:

- ***Weight Gain and Metabolism:*** Elevated cortisol levels signal the body to store fat, especially around the abdominal area. This is because the body perceives chronic stress as a survival mechanism, which requires energy stores. The long-term result can be stubborn belly fat that is hard to lose. Cortisol also interferes with insulin sensitivity, making it more difficult for the body to regulate blood sugar levels, which can lead to weight gain.

- ***Sleep Disruption:*** Cortisol is a natural regulator of your sleep-wake cycle, known as the circadian rhythm. Normally, cortisol levels drop at night to help you sleep, and rise in the morning to help you wake up. However, when stress levels are high, cortisol remains elevated at night, making it difficult to fall and stay asleep. This contributes to insomnia, poor-quality sleep, and daytime fatigue.

- *Mood and Mental Health:* Chronic high cortisol can negatively impact your mood, leading to increased feelings of anxiety, irritability, and even depression. It can also impair cognitive function, reducing memory and concentration. Cortisol suppresses the production of serotonin, the "feel-good" hormone, which contributes to mood disorders.

- *Immune System Suppression:* While cortisol helps control inflammation, excessive cortisol can suppress the immune system, making your body more susceptible to illness and infection. Over time, this can lead to chronic health conditions, autoimmune diseases, and a slower recovery from injury or illness.

- *Hormonal Imbalance:* Cortisol is closely linked to other hormones in the body, including thyroid hormones, insulin, and reproductive hormones. When cortisol is out of balance, it can disrupt the function of these other hormones, leading to further health problems such as thyroid dysfunction, insulin resistance, and menstrual irregularities.

The Modern Epidemic: Stress and Hormonal Imbalance

In today's fast-paced world, stress is virtually unavoidable. From work deadlines and financial concerns to personal relationships and societal pressures, the modern world bombards us with constant stressors. With the constant demands on our time and attention, our bodies are in a state of near-perpetual stress, leading to elevated cortisol levels that can go on for days, weeks, months, and even years.

Unfortunately, many people are unaware of how deeply stress is affecting their bodies. Most individuals only become aware of the consequences when they experience the physical and emotional effects: unexplained weight gain, insomnia, anxiety, fatigue, or difficulty concentrating. These symptoms are often mistakenly attributed to aging or simply a result of living in a demanding world, but in reality, they are the direct consequences of chronic cortisol imbalance.

Over time, this ongoing stress not only wears down your body's resilience but can lead to a host of chronic conditions, including:

- *Heart disease*
- *Type 2 diabetes*
- *Digestive problems*
- *High blood pressure*
- *Hormonal disorders*

It's no wonder that stress has been called a silent killer. It may not manifest in a single catastrophic event, but it chips away at your health, slowly diminishing your quality of life.

How This Book Will Transform Your Life

Now that you understand cortisol's vital role in your health and well-being, you may be wondering, "What can I do about it?" The good news is that you have the power to take control of your cortisol levels and begin the journey toward restoring balance in your body. The strategies, tools, and meal plans provided in this book will guide you step-by-step on how to detox from cortisol overload and improve your overall health.

This book is more than just a diet guide—it's a comprehensive plan for healing your body and mind. Here's how this book will help you transform your life:

- ***Reset Your Hormones:*** By following the cortisol detox principles, you'll be able to naturally lower cortisol levels in your body, restoring balance to your hormones. This process will allow your body to function optimally, leading to improved sleep, better energy levels, reduced inflammation, and a stronger immune system.
- ***Achieve Sustainable Weight Loss:*** As you regulate cortisol levels, you'll find it easier to lose stubborn belly fat and keep it off. The meal plans and recipes in this book are designed to support healthy metabolism and promote fat loss without feeling deprived or stressed about food.
- ***Experience Mental Clarity:*** Lowering cortisol will not only improve your physical health, but it will also help you feel more relaxed and focused. Say goodbye to constant brain fog, anxiety, and stress, and welcome a clearer, calmer mind.

*- **Reclaim Your Health and Happiness:*** The cortisol detox diet plan is about more than just physical appearance—it's about healing your body and mind. By following this plan, you'll feel energized, balanced, and empowered to take on life with renewed vitality. The transformation will leave you feeling more confident, less stressed, and more at peace.

*- **Develop Healthy Habits for Life:*** This book is designed to be a lifelong solution. Once you understand the principles of cortisol management and detoxing, you'll be able to integrate these practices into your daily routine. The diet, stress reduction techniques, and lifestyle changes outlined in this book are not just quick fixes—they are sustainable habits that will continue to improve your health long-term.

A Holistic Approach to Wellness

This book takes a holistic approach to wellness, meaning that it addresses the root causes of cortisol imbalance and offers comprehensive solutions. Through diet, exercise, mindfulness practices, and stress management techniques, you will learn how to treat the underlying stress that's causing your cortisol levels to rise. With practical steps and easy-to-follow meal plans, this book will help you build a healthier, more balanced life.

You will begin by learning about the role cortisol plays in your body, how to recognize the signs of hormonal imbalance, and how stress affects your physical and mental health. From there, you'll dive into the step-by-step strategies to detox cortisol from your system, supported by a 21-day meal plan filled with delicious, easy-to-make recipes that will support your health and help you feel your best.

CHAPTER 2

Understanding Cortisol

The Science Behind Cortisol: A Deep Dive

Cortisol is a steroid hormone that is produced by the adrenal glands, which sit atop your kidneys. It's often referred to as the "stress hormone" because its primary function is to help your body respond to stress. However, cortisol is involved in many other processes and is essential for normal body function. Let's explore the complex biology of cortisol and how it impacts your health.

The Cortisol Production Process

Cortisol is released into the bloodstream through a process known as the hypothalamic-pituitary-adrenal (HPA) axis, which involves three key players:

1. The Hypothalamus: Located in the brain, this part of your nervous system is responsible for sensing stress and releasing signals that activate the other two components.

2. The Pituitary Gland: Once the hypothalamus detects stress, it signals the pituitary gland to release adrenocorticotropic hormone (ACTH), which stimulates the adrenal glands to produce cortisol.

3. The Adrenal Glands: These small glands release cortisol into the bloodstream. Once it's released, cortisol circulates throughout the body, reaching various organs and tissues, where it has multiple physiological effects.

The Role of Cortisol in Stress Response

When your body faces stress (such as a physical injury, emotional trauma, or a stressful work situation), cortisol is released as part of the "fight or flight" response. Cortisol helps to:

- *Increase glucose levels:* This provides immediate energy for your muscles and brain, helping you react quickly.

- *Boost alertness:* Cortisol enhances focus and mental clarity during stressful situations.

- *Regulate inflammation:* Cortisol suppresses inflammation to prevent the body from overreacting to stress.

- Manage blood pressure: Cortisol helps maintain blood pressure by controlling sodium balance and regulating blood vessels.

While cortisol is essential for handling short-term stress, its role in chronic, long-term stress is much more complex. When cortisol remains elevated for extended periods, it can have negative effects on the body, particularly when combined with lifestyle factors like poor diet, lack of exercise, and insufficient sleep.

Signs of High Cortisol Levels

Chronic stress leads to consistently high levels of cortisol, which can manifest in a variety of physical, emotional, and mental symptoms. Here are some of the most common signs of elevated cortisol levels:

Physical Symptoms:

1. Abdominal Fat Storage: One of the hallmarks of high cortisol levels is the accumulation of fat around the abdominal area. This is because cortisol prompts the body to store fat as an energy reserve for stress. The abdominal region, often referred to as "visceral fat," is particularly vulnerable to cortisol-induced fat storage.

2. Fatigue and Exhaustion: Ironically, while cortisol is meant to boost energy, chronic high cortisol can lead to fatigue and exhaustion. This happens because your adrenal glands become overworked and struggle to produce other vital hormones, leading to feelings of burnout.

3. Frequent Illnesses: Because cortisol suppresses the immune system over time, elevated cortisol can lead to frequent colds, infections, or slower recovery from illness. Chronic inflammation, which is associated with high cortisol, also weakens immune function.

4. Digestive Issues: High cortisol levels are associated with gut imbalances, causing symptoms like bloating, indigestion, heartburn, and irritable bowel syndrome (IBS). Cortisol also affects the gut microbiome, potentially leading to an increase in harmful bacteria and a decrease in beneficial bacteria.

5. Headaches: Cortisol is linked to changes in blood flow and inflammation in the body, which can lead to tension headaches or migraines. These types of headaches are more common in individuals with prolonged stress.

<u>**Emotional and Mental Symptoms:**</u>

1. Mood Swings and Irritability: High cortisol levels are directly related to emotional instability. When cortisol is chronically elevated, it can lead to feelings of anxiety, irritability, and mood swings. This is because cortisol suppresses serotonin and other neurotransmitters that regulate mood.

2. Anxiety and Depression: Constantly high cortisol levels can interfere with the brain's ability to regulate emotions, which increases the risk of developing mood disorders like anxiety and depression. Elevated cortisol levels contribute to the dysregulation of the limbic system, which controls emotions and stress responses.

3. Memory and Focus Issues: Cortisol has a direct effect on brain function, particularly in areas like memory, focus, and learning. Chronic stress and high cortisol levels are associated with impaired cognitive function and memory recall. Over time, this can lead to a phenomenon known as "brain fog," where you struggle to concentrate and remember important information.

4. Sleep Problems: High cortisol levels interfere with your body's natural circadian rhythm. Cortisol is usually highest in the morning, helping you wake up and feel alert, but in individuals with high chronic cortisol, the hormone may stay elevated at night, preventing deep sleep and causing insomnia. This leads to a cycle of exhaustion and poor sleep quality.

The Impact of Cortisol on Weight, Sleep, and Mood

Cortisol's impact on the body extends far beyond its role in stress response. The hormone plays a critical role in regulating key processes like metabolism, sleep, and emotional well-being. Let's take a closer look at how cortisol affects weight, sleep, and mood:

<u>**Cortisol and Weight**</u>

As mentioned earlier, cortisol is a key factor in fat storage, especially around the abdominal region. Here's how cortisol affects weight:

1. Increased Appetite and Cravings: Elevated cortisol levels can increase hunger, particularly cravings for sugary and fatty foods. This is because cortisol stimulates the release of insulin, which helps to store energy in the form of fat. When insulin levels rise in response to stress, your body craves quick sources of energy, like carbohydrates, which can lead to overeating.

2. Fat Storage: Cortisol directly promotes fat storage, particularly in the belly area. This is a survival mechanism, as the body believes it needs to store fat for energy during times of stress. Unfortunately, the body doesn't differentiate between real danger (like running from a tiger) and perceived stress (like a difficult work situation), leading to fat accumulation in the abdominal region.

3. Muscle Breakdown: High cortisol levels can also lead to muscle breakdown. When cortisol levels remain elevated for long periods, the body starts breaking down muscle tissue for energy. This leads to muscle loss, which in turn slows down your metabolism and makes it harder to burn fat.

Cortisol and Sleep

Sleep is one of the most important aspects of health, and cortisol plays a central role in regulating the sleep-wake cycle. High cortisol levels can disrupt sleep in several ways:

1. Delayed Sleep Onset: Elevated cortisol levels can make it harder to fall asleep at night. Cortisol usually peaks in the morning and drops in the evening to prepare the body for sleep, but when stress is chronic, cortisol can remain high at night, preventing the body from transitioning into a restful sleep state.

2. Poor Sleep Quality: Even if you manage to fall asleep, high cortisol levels can lead to poor sleep quality, including frequent waking, restless sleep, and reduced time spent in the restorative stages of sleep (such as deep sleep). This contributes to feelings of fatigue and low energy the next day.

3. Sleep Disorders: Prolonged high cortisol levels are linked to sleep disorders like insomnia and sleep apnea. These disorders disrupt the natural circadian rhythm, making it even harder for the body to recover and regenerate during sleep.

Cortisol and Mood

Your mood is heavily influenced by cortisol. Here's how cortisol affects emotional well-being:

1. Increased Anxiety and Stress: Chronic cortisol release can elevate feelings of anxiety and stress. When cortisol remains elevated over time, it can overwhelm the body's ability to cope with stress, leading to feelings of constant worry, tension, and unease.

2. Depression and Fatigue: Cortisol is involved in regulating neurotransmitters like serotonin and dopamine, which are essential for maintaining a balanced mood.

High cortisol levels suppress these neurotransmitters, which can lead to feelings of depression, low energy, and emotional numbness.

3. Cognitive Impairment: High cortisol levels can impair cognitive functions such as memory, focus, and learning. This leads to problems with concentration, mental clarity, and overall cognitive performance, contributing to feelings of frustration and self-doubt.

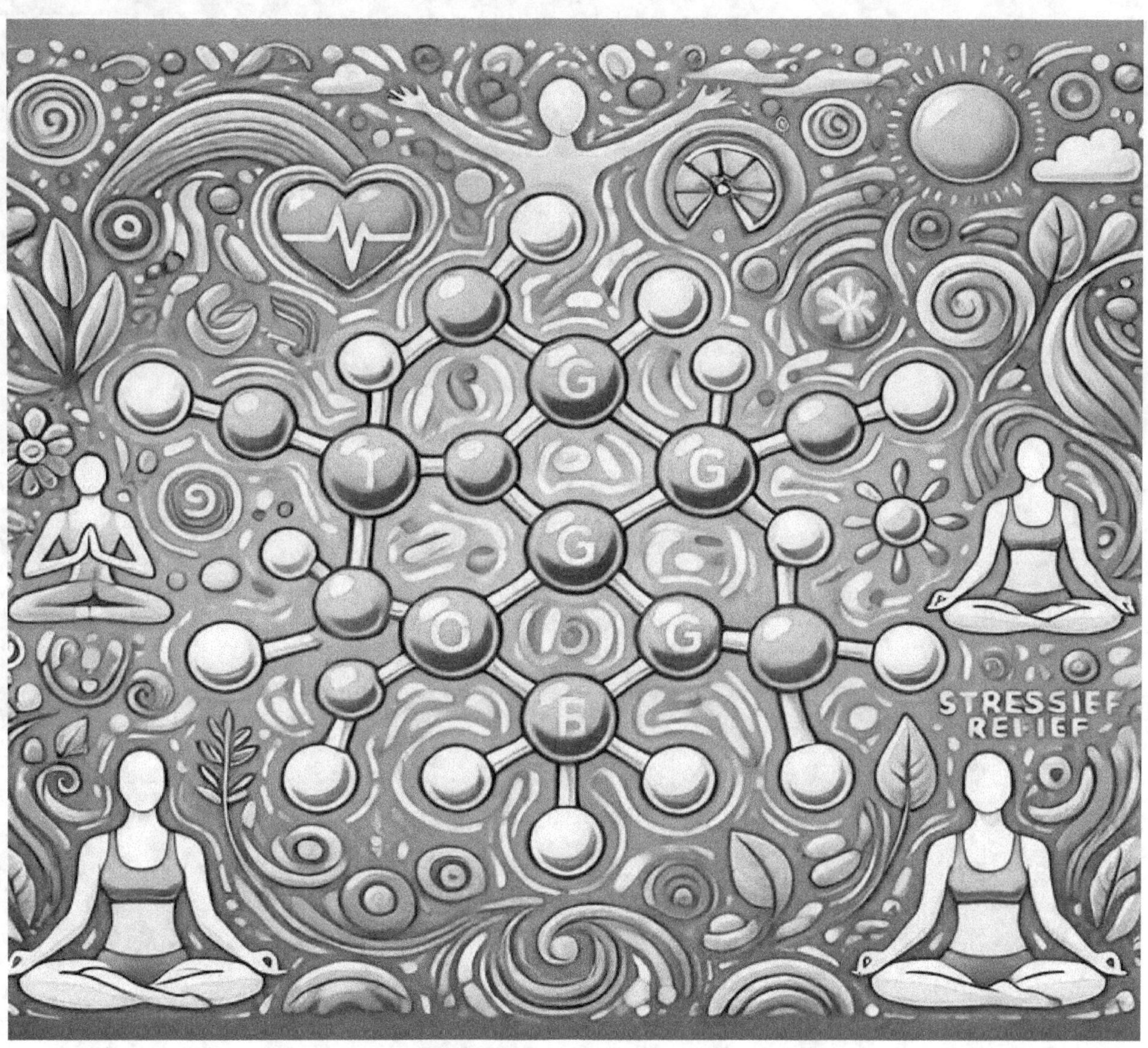

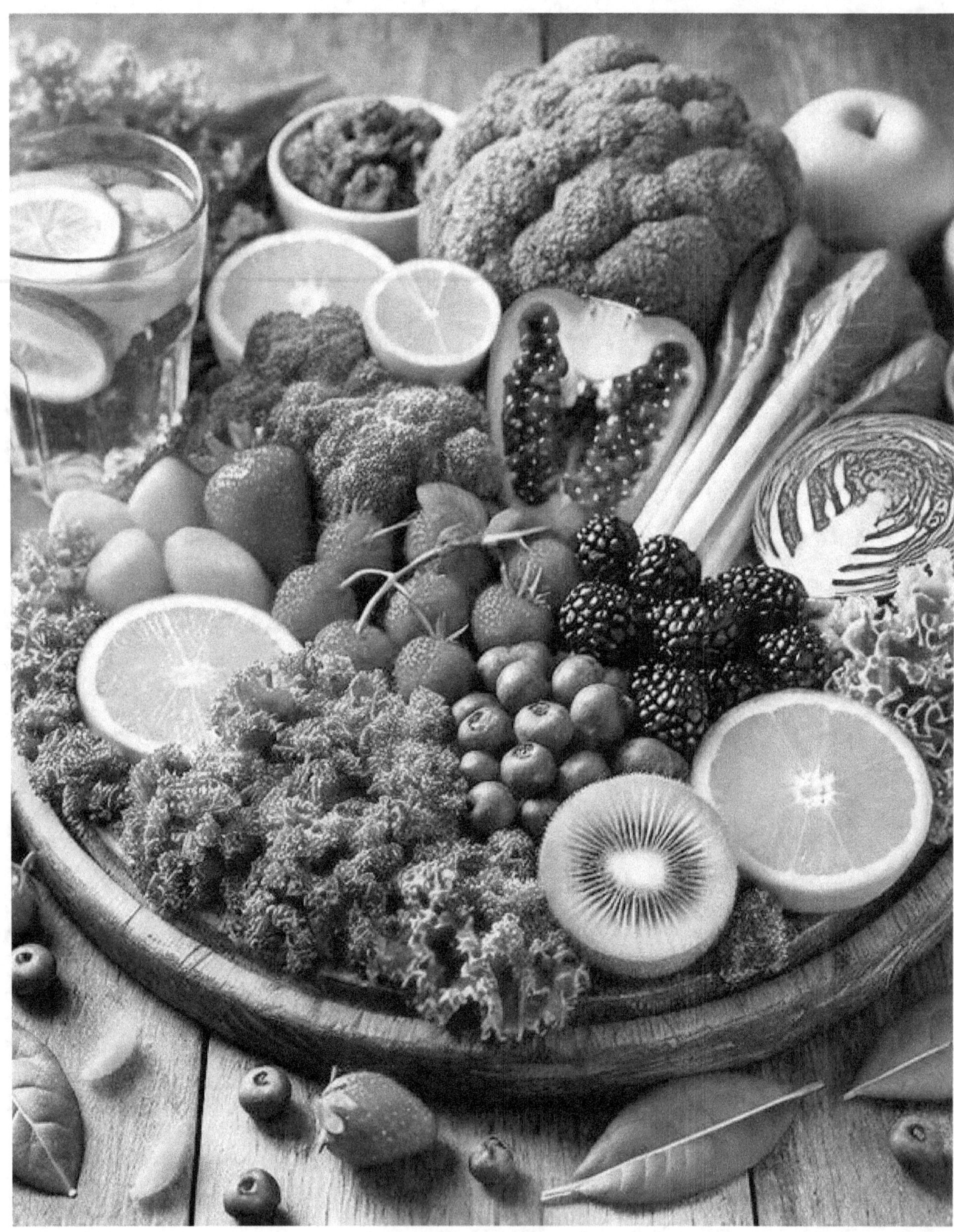

CHAPTER 3

The Detox Solution

Why Detoxing Works

Detoxing has been a popular concept in the health and wellness community for years, but what makes it such an effective strategy? Detoxing is not just about "cleansing" the body of toxins, but about giving the body the support it needs to restore balance, optimize its functions, and regain control over the factors that contribute to cortisol imbalance. Let's break down why detoxing works, especially in relation to cortisol management.

1. Reducing Toxins and Inflammation: Chronic stress, poor diet, and environmental factors contribute to the build-up of toxins and inflammation in the body. These toxins, often stored in the liver, kidneys, and fat cells, can create imbalances in your hormones, including cortisol. By detoxing, you remove these harmful substances, allowing the body to function more efficiently. The reduction of inflammation and toxins helps lower cortisol production, which in turn alleviates stress and promotes a balanced hormonal environment.

2. Supporting Liver Function: The liver plays a critical role in detoxification, as it filters out waste products and toxins from the bloodstream. When the liver is overloaded or sluggish due to poor eating habits, excessive alcohol consumption, or environmental toxins, it cannot properly process cortisol or other hormones. Detoxing encourages the liver to function optimally, supporting the removal of excess cortisol and other waste products. A well-functioning liver ensures that cortisol levels are better regulated, reducing the body's overall stress burden.

3. Restoring Nutrient Balance: The modern diet is often nutrient-deficient, lacking vital vitamins and minerals that help regulate cortisol levels. A detox plan introduces nutrient-dense foods that promote hormonal balance and overall well-being. For example, foods rich in magnesium, B vitamins, and vitamin C help reduce cortisol production and support the adrenal glands in managing stress. Detoxing is not about extreme calorie restriction or deprivation; it's about providing the body with the tools it needs to reset and thrive.

4. Enhancing Gut Health: Gut health and cortisol levels are closely linked. The gut is home to trillions of bacteria that influence everything from digestion to immunity, and even mood regulation. When the gut is unbalanced, it can trigger an inflammatory response that elevates cortisol. Detoxing supports the gut by introducing fiber-rich foods, prebiotics, and probiotics that restore balance to the microbiome. A healthy gut promotes optimal cortisol regulation and helps to manage stress better.

5. *Reducing Stress on the Body:* Cortisol is released in response to stress, and when your body is overloaded with toxins, poor nutrition, and insufficient sleep, it perceives these as threats, thereby triggering more cortisol production. Detoxing offers a chance to reset your body and mind, reducing the physical and mental stress that leads to chronic cortisol imbalance. By addressing the root causes of stress, detoxing helps your body regain its natural rhythm and reduces the constant flood of cortisol.

In essence, detoxing works because it provides the body with an opportunity to reset, heal, and recalibrate. It's not just about eliminating toxins—it's about creating the optimal environment for balanced hormones, improved energy, and a calmer, more resilient body.

The Cortisol Detox Blueprint: 7 Core Principles

The Cortisol Detox Blueprint is designed to guide you through a step-by-step process for lowering cortisol levels and restoring balance to your body. This holistic approach combines diet, lifestyle changes, and mindfulness practices to help you achieve lasting results. Here are the seven core principles that form the foundation of the Cortisol Detox Blueprint:

1. *Cleanse and Nourish Your Body with Whole Foods:* The first step in the blueprint is to nourish your body with whole, unprocessed foods that are rich in nutrients, antioxidants, and fiber. These foods support the liver, kidneys, and digestive system, enabling them to detoxify the body more effectively. Focus on consuming:
  - *Fresh vegetables and fruits:* These provide vitamins, minerals, and antioxidants that help lower inflammation.
  - *Healthy fats:* Omega-3 fatty acids from sources like avocados, nuts, seeds, and oily fish support brain function and reduce cortisol production.

- *Lean proteins:* Protein-rich foods help maintain muscle mass, stabilize blood sugar, and provide sustained energy, reducing stress.

2. *Hydrate for Detoxification:* Water is essential for detoxification as it helps flush toxins from the body, supports the kidneys, and promotes healthy circulation. Staying hydrated also supports digestion, reduces hunger cravings, and helps balance cortisol levels. Aim to drink at least 8-10 glasses of water daily, and incorporate herbal teas like chamomile, dandelion, or ginger, which have detoxifying and stress-reducing properties.

3. *Prioritize Gut Health:* A healthy gut is essential for cortisol regulation. The gut-brain connection plays a significant role in the release of stress hormones, including cortisol. To support gut health during your detox:

- Include prebiotic and probiotic foods such as garlic, onions, bananas, yogurt, kefir, sauerkraut, and kimchi.
- Avoid processed foods, sugar, and refined carbohydrates, which can harm the gut microbiome and increase cortisol levels.
- Consider incorporating digestive enzymes or herbal teas like peppermint to soothe and support digestion.

4. *Engage in Stress-Reducing Activities:* Cortisol is primarily a stress hormone, so managing stress is crucial for your detox success. The blueprint encourages the use of relaxation techniques and mindfulness practices to reduce stress and calm the nervous system. Some effective stress-reducing practices include:

- *Meditation:* Just 10-15 minutes of meditation per day can reduce cortisol levels and improve emotional well-being.
- *Yoga:* Gentle movement and breathing exercises help calm the body and mind, promoting relaxation and balance.
- *Breathing exercises:* Techniques like deep belly breathing can lower cortisol and activate the parasympathetic nervous system, which helps the body relax.

5. *Get Quality Sleep:* Sleep is one of the most powerful tools for reducing cortisol. When you don't get enough restorative sleep, cortisol levels spike, and your body remains in a state of stress. To enhance sleep quality during your detox:

- Establish a consistent bedtime routine to signal to your body that it's time to wind down.
- Limit exposure to blue light from screens before bed and create a peaceful environment conducive to sleep.

- Try using relaxing scents such as lavender, chamomile, or sandalwood in your bedroom to promote calmness.

6. Exercise to Regulate Cortisol: Exercise is a powerful tool for balancing cortisol levels, but it's important to find the right balance. Overtraining or intense exercise can increase cortisol, while moderate exercise helps manage it. The key is to focus on:

- Moderate, low-impact exercises such as walking, swimming, and cycling.
- Incorporate strength training to build muscle and improve metabolism, which helps regulate cortisol.
- Try mindful movement practices like tai chi or yoga to reduce stress and enhance relaxation.

7. Avoid Stimulants and Toxins: During your detox, it's essential to minimize the intake of substances that trigger cortisol production, such as caffeine, alcohol, and processed foods. These stimulants can elevate cortisol levels and interfere with your body's natural detoxification process. Instead, choose:

- Herbal teas like lemon balm, valerian root, or passionflower, which have calming effects.
- Whole foods and antioxidant-rich foods that help neutralize toxins and support detoxification.

These seven principles form the core of the Cortisol Detox Blueprint, giving you the tools to reset your body, lower cortisol, and improve your overall health. The blueprint is designed to be adaptable, so you can incorporate it into your lifestyle at your own pace while achieving optimal results.

Preparing Your Body for Success

Before you embark on your cortisol detox journey, it's essential to prepare your body and mind for success. Successful detoxification requires commitment, consistency, and a willingness to make positive changes. Here's how you can prepare for the transformation ahead:

1. Clean Up Your Environment: Remove any unhealthy food, beverages, or stressors from your home environment. Clear out junk food, processed snacks, and sugary drinks that may tempt you to fall back into old habits. Stock your kitchen with nourishing foods, herbal teas, and other detox-friendly items that support your journey.

2. Set Clear Goals and Intentions: Be clear about why you are undertaking this detox. Whether your goal is to lower cortisol, improve sleep, lose weight, or enhance your mood, setting clear and realistic goals will help you stay focused and motivated throughout the process.

3. Take a Mindful Approach: Your mindset plays a huge role in your success. Approach the detox process with patience, compassion, and mindfulness. There may be challenges along the way, but remember that detoxing is a gradual process, and every small step brings you closer to a balanced, cortisol-free body.

4. Monitor Your Progress: Track your progress throughout the detox to stay accountable and motivated. Record your sleep patterns, stress levels, weight, and any physical or emotional changes you experience. This will help you assess how your body is responding and make any necessary adjustments along the way.

By preparing your body, setting clear intentions, and following the Cortisol Detox Blueprint, you can create the foundation for long-term success in managing cortisol levels and achieving a healthier, more balanced life.

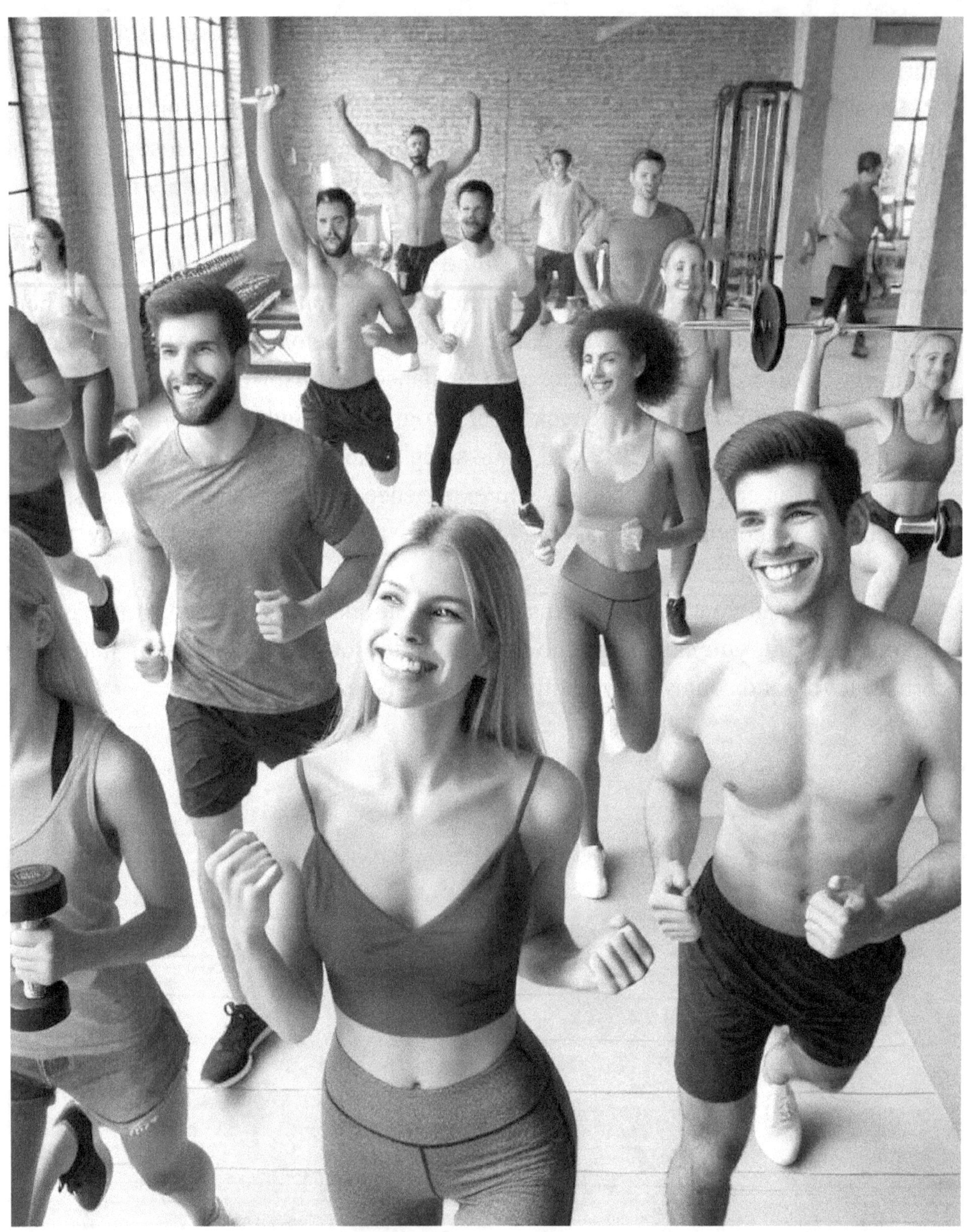

CHAPTER 4

The Cortisol Detox Diet Plan

Recipes and Strategies

Embarking on the Cortisol Detox Diet Plan can be a transformative experience, and one of the most effective ways to reset your body and balance cortisol is through a structured, nutrient-rich meal plan. This 21-day detox meal plan is designed to help reduce stress, nourish your body, and support your adrenal glands, all while incorporating foods that naturally lower cortisol levels. During this detox, it's also important to incorporate self-care practices such as meditation, journaling, and gentle exercise.

Best Foods to Balance Cortisol Levels

The foods you eat play a significant role in regulating cortisol. When it comes to balancing cortisol, your diet should include nutrient-dense, anti-inflammatory foods that support overall health and stabilize your body's stress response. Here are some of the best foods to balance cortisol:

1. Omega-3 Fatty Acids: Omega-3 fatty acids are known for their ability to reduce inflammation and support brain health. These fats help lower cortisol levels and can be found in:
- Fatty fish (salmon, mackerel, sardines)
- Walnuts
- Flaxseeds and chia seeds
- Hemp seeds

2. Leafy Greens: Leafy greens like spinach, kale, and Swiss chard are packed with magnesium, a mineral that helps regulate cortisol and relax the muscles. Magnesium-rich foods help your body adapt to stress and can prevent spikes in cortisol.

3. Berries: Berries like blueberries, strawberries, and raspberries are full of antioxidants, which help reduce inflammation and oxidative stress in the body. Antioxidants fight free radicals that trigger cortisol production, promoting hormonal balance.

4. *Avocados:* Avocados are rich in healthy fats and potassium, both of which are vital for reducing cortisol and supporting overall health. The monounsaturated fats in avocados also help keep blood sugar levels stable, reducing cortisol spikes.

5. *Herbal Teas:* Herbal teas such as chamomile, lemon balm, and ashwagandha are known for their calming and stress-reducing properties. They help lower cortisol levels and promote relaxation, making them an ideal choice for managing stress.

6. *Adaptogenic Herbs:* Adaptogens are herbs that help the body cope with stress and maintain hormonal balance. Some popular adaptogens include:
- *Ashwagandha:* Known to reduce cortisol levels and improve sleep.
- *Rhodiola:* Enhances the body's resilience to stress.
- *Holy basil:* Supports the adrenal glands and reduces the effects of chronic stress.

7. *Sweet Potatoes and Root Vegetables:* Sweet potatoes and other root vegetables are rich in complex carbohydrates and fiber. These foods help stabilize blood sugar levels, preventing spikes in cortisol. They also provide a steady source of energy to the body.

8. *Dark Chocolate:* Dark chocolate (with at least 70% cocoa) is not only a delicious treat but also a stress-reducing food. It contains flavonoids and magnesium, which can lower cortisol and improve mood. Just be sure to consume it in moderation.

9. *Probiotic-Rich Foods:* Probiotics help promote gut health, which is closely connected to stress and cortisol regulation. Foods like yogurt, kefir, kimchi, and sauerkraut contain beneficial bacteria that support digestion and help lower cortisol levels.

10. *Whole Grains:* Whole grains such as quinoa, brown rice, and oats are rich in fiber and B vitamins, which support adrenal function and lower cortisol. They also stabilize blood sugar levels, reducing stress-induced cortisol spikes.

By incorporating these foods into your diet, you can create a balanced and sustainable approach to managing cortisol levels while nourishing your body with essential nutrients.

Hydration and Herbal Support

In addition to eating a balanced diet, staying hydrated and incorporating herbal support are essential for reducing cortisol levels. Here's how hydration and herbal support play a vital role in the detox process:

- ***Hydration:*** Water is essential for detoxification, as it helps flush out toxins, supports kidney function, and regulates cortisol production. Dehydration is a stressor on the body and can lead to increased cortisol levels. Be sure to drink at least 8-10 glasses of water daily to stay hydrated. You can also drink coconut water, which is rich in electrolytes and helps balance cortisol.
- ***Herbal Support:*** Herbs can provide significant support during your detox process by reducing stress, improving sleep quality, and promoting hormone balance. Some beneficial herbs to include in your daily routine are:
    - *Chamomile:* Calms the nervous system and improves sleep.
    - *Ashwagandha:* A powerful adaptogen that helps manage stress and balance cortisol.
    - *Lemon balm:* Reduces anxiety and promotes relaxation.
    - *Rhodiola:* Enhances energy, reduces fatigue, and lowers cortisol as earlier mentioned.
    - *Holy basil:* Helps the body cope with stress and reduces cortisol production.

Drinking herbal teas or incorporating these herbs into your daily routine can offer additional support for reducing cortisol and optimizing your detox process.

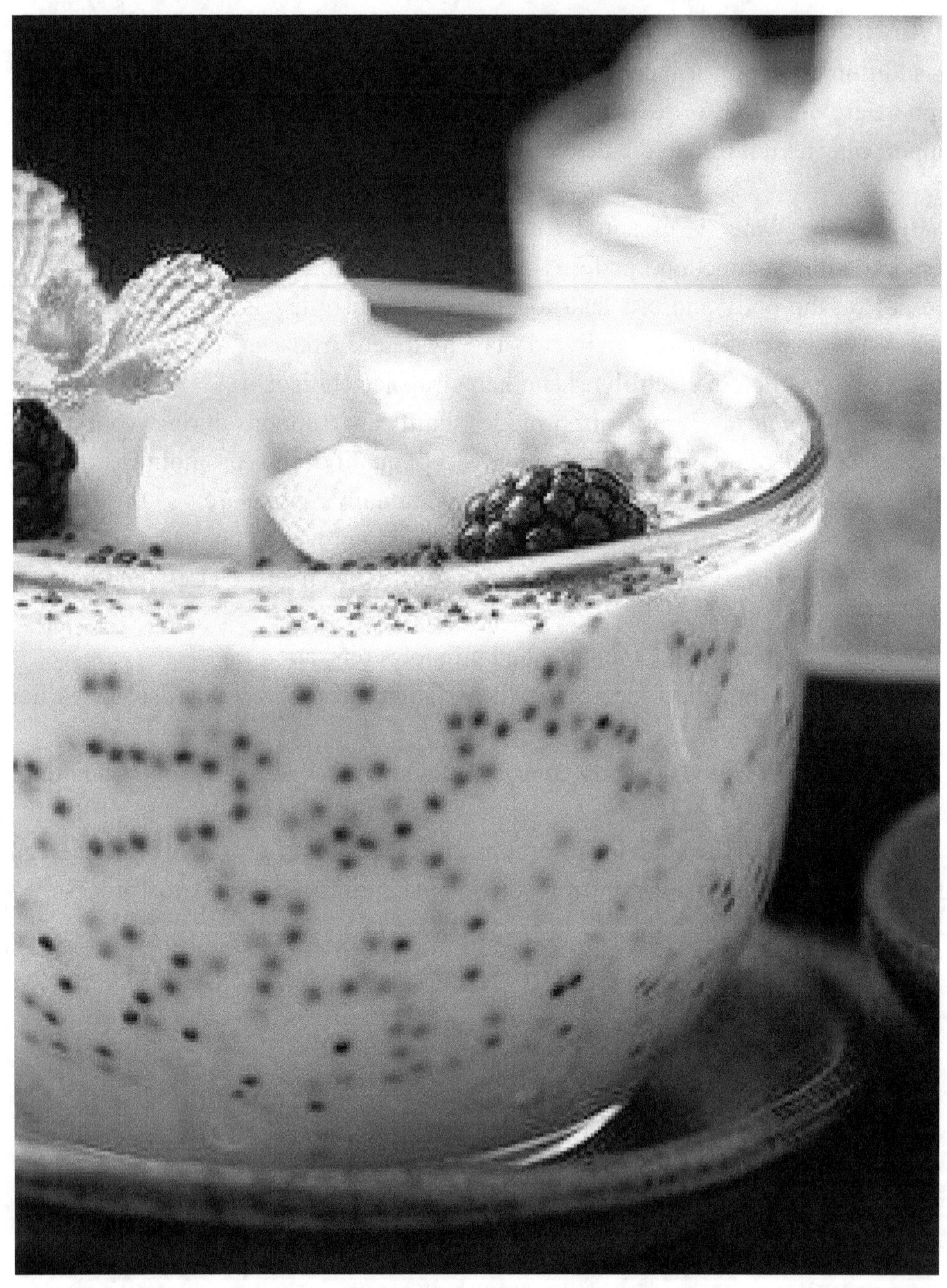

CHAPTER 5

Lifestyle Changes for Lasting Results

While diet plays a pivotal role in lowering cortisol levels, lifestyle changes are just as essential to ensure that the results from your Cortisol Detox Diet Plan are sustainable in the long term. Stress management, sleep hygiene, and mindfulness practices can help you maintain a balanced cortisol level, optimize your hormonal health, and enhance overall well-being. In this chapter, we'll explore practical, evidence-based techniques to help you achieve lasting results.

Stress Management Techniques That Work

Chronic stress is one of the leading causes of elevated cortisol levels. To achieve lasting hormonal balance, it's important to incorporate effective stress management techniques into your daily routine. These strategies will help you reduce the stressors in your life, manage those you can't avoid, and support your body in maintaining calmness and resilience.

1. Breathing Exercises: Deep, intentional breathing helps activate the parasympathetic nervous system (your "rest and digest" system), which lowers cortisol and promotes relaxation. Here are some simple breathing exercises that can quickly reduce stress and lower cortisol:

- *Box Breathing (Square Breathing):* Inhale for 4 counts, hold for 4 counts, exhale for 4 counts, and hold for 4 counts. Repeat for several minutes to activate your parasympathetic nervous system.
- *4-7-8 Breathing:* Inhale for 4 counts, hold for 7 counts, and exhale for 8 counts. This deep breathing exercise calms the nervous system and reduces cortisol.

2. Physical Activity: Regular physical activity is one of the most powerful tools for reducing stress and lowering cortisol. It helps release endorphins (the body's natural "feel-good" chemicals), improves mood, and reduces anxiety. However, it's essential to find a balance between exercise and rest, as over-exercising can actually increase cortisol levels.

- *Moderate Exercise:* Walking, yoga, cycling, and swimming can all help reduce cortisol without over-stressing your body.

- *Mindful Movement:* Activities like yoga, tai chi, or Pilates combine gentle movement with focused breathing, which reduces both physical and mental stress.

*3. **Time in Nature:*** Spending time outdoors has been shown to significantly reduce stress and lower cortisol levels. Even short walks in a park or forest can have a profound effect on your body's stress response. The natural environment helps promote a sense of calm and connectedness, which can balance hormones and improve overall mental health.

*4. **Journaling:*** Writing down your thoughts, worries, or reflections can be a highly effective way of managing stress. Journaling helps clear your mind, release pent-up emotions, and bring perspective to your thoughts. This practice is particularly useful for processing stress or anxiety, which can lead to higher cortisol levels.

*5. **Social Support and Connection:*** Strong social connections and spending time with loved ones can reduce stress and enhance well-being. Whether it's sharing a laugh with friends, enjoying a conversation with family, or seeking professional support, fostering healthy relationships helps buffer the effects of stress on your body.

The Power of Sleep in Hormonal Health

Sleep is not only essential for physical health, but it is also one of the most important factors in balancing cortisol and maintaining a healthy hormonal system. Poor sleep or sleep deprivation can lead to an imbalance in cortisol levels, causing them to spike during the night and preventing your body from properly recovering and resetting.

*1. **The Sleep-Cortisol Connection:*** Cortisol follows a natural rhythm called the diurnal rhythm, which means that it peaks in the morning to help you wake up and decreases throughout the day, reaching its lowest point at night. However, poor sleep can disrupt this cycle, causing cortisol levels to remain elevated when they should be decreasing.

When you get sufficient and quality sleep, your body has the time it needs to repair itself and restore balance to your hormones. Sleep deprivation, on the other hand, can lead to an increase in cortisol production, which can disrupt the sleep cycle, leading to a vicious cycle of stress and sleeplessness.

2. Sleep Hygiene Tips: To ensure quality sleep and support your cortisol levels, it's important to establish a consistent and restorative sleep routine. Here are some practical tips to improve your sleep hygiene:

- *Create a Sleep Schedule:* Go to bed and wake up at the same time each day, even on weekends, to regulate your body's internal clock.
- *Limit Blue Light Exposure:* Avoid screens (phones, computers, TVs) at least 30 minutes to an hour before bed, as the blue light emitted from screens can interfere with melatonin production and delay sleep.
- *Set a Relaxing Bedtime Routine:* Consider incorporating calming activities like reading, taking a warm bath, or practicing gentle stretches before bed to signal to your body that it's time to wind down.
- *Create an Optimal Sleep Environment:* Keep your bedroom cool, quiet, and dark to create the ideal environment for sleep. Consider using blackout curtains, earplugs, or a white noise machine if needed.
- *Limit Caffeine and Alcohol:* Avoid caffeine at least 6 hours before bedtime, as it can interfere with sleep quality. Similarly, while alcohol may initially make you feel drowsy, it disrupts deep sleep cycles and can elevate cortisol during the night.

3. The Role of Napping: Short, controlled naps can provide a significant energy boost and reduce stress without negatively affecting nighttime sleep. Keep naps to 20–30 minutes to avoid disrupting your body's natural sleep-wake cycle. Avoid napping late in the day to prevent it from interfering with your nighttime rest.

Mindfulness and Meditation: A Daily Practice

Mindfulness and meditation are powerful tools for reducing stress and lowering cortisol levels. By practicing mindfulness, you can learn to observe your thoughts and emotions without becoming overwhelmed by them, which helps create mental clarity and emotional balance. Meditation, on the other hand, provides a structured approach to calming your mind, lowering stress, and promoting relaxation.

1. The Science Behind Mindfulness: Mindfulness practices have been shown to reduce cortisol and improve emotional regulation. Research indicates that mindfulness can lower anxiety, reduce the effects of stress, and help regulate the body's response to negative emotions. Regular mindfulness practice can also improve sleep quality, enhance cognitive function, and reduce symptoms of depression.

2. Meditation Techniques: There are various types of meditation that can help reduce cortisol levels, including:

- *Guided Meditation:* Follow along with a recorded meditation that guides you through breathing exercises and visualizations. Apps like Calm or Headspace can provide structured meditation sessions tailored to your needs.
- *Loving-Kindness Meditation:* This practice focuses on cultivating feelings of compassion and love toward yourself and others, which can help soften stress and improve your emotional resilience.
- *Body Scan Meditation:* A technique that involves mentally scanning each part of your body from head to toe, promoting relaxation and reducing tension.

3. How to Incorporate Mindfulness into Daily Life: You don't need to set aside hours each day for mindfulness or meditation. Here are some simple ways to integrate mindfulness into your daily routine:

- *Mindful Breathing:* Take a few moments throughout your day to focus on your breath. Inhale deeply and slowly, paying attention to how your body feels with each breath. This simple practice can calm your nervous system and reduce cortisol.
- *Mindful Eating:* Slow down and savor each bite of food, paying full attention to the textures, flavors, and aromas. This practice not only promotes digestion but also helps you reduce stress and feel more present.
- *Mindful Walking:* Whether you're walking outside or simply moving through your home, practice being fully aware of your movements and the sensations in your body. Notice the sounds, smells, and sights around you.

CHAPTER 6

Recipes for Hormonal Harmony

Breakfast: Energizing Morning Meals

1. Stress-Busting Green Smoothie Bowl

Cook time: 5 mins / Prep time: 5 mins / Serves: 1

INGREDIENTS:
- 1/2 cup spinach
- 1/2 banana
- 1/4 avocado
- 1/2 cup almond milk
- 1 tbsp chia seeds
- 1 tsp spirulina powder (optional)
- 1/4 cup granola
- 1 tbsp almond butter

INSTRUCTIONS:
1. Blend spinach, banana, avocado, almond milk, chia seeds, and spirulina powder until smooth.
2. Pour into a bowl and top with granola and almond butter.
3. Enjoy immediately!

NUTRITIONAL INFORMATION (per serving):
- Calories: 320
- Protein: 7g
- Carbs: 30g
- Fat: 18g
- Fiber: 10g

2. Overnight Chia Pudding with Berries

Cook time: 0 mins / Prep time: 10 mins / Serves: 2

INGREDIENTS:

- 1/2 cup chia seeds
- 1 cup almond milk
- 1 tbsp maple syrup
- 1/2 tsp vanilla extract
- 1/4 cup mixed berries (blueberries, raspberries, strawberries)
- 1 tbsp sliced almonds

INSTRUCTIONS:

1. In a bowl or jar, mix chia seeds, almond milk, maple syrup, and vanilla extract.
2. Stir to combine and let sit for 5 minutes.
3. Cover and refrigerate overnight.
4. In the morning, stir and top with mixed berries and sliced almonds.

NUTRITIONAL INFORMATION (per serving):

- Calories: 280
- Protein: 8g
- Carbs: 24g
- Fat: 18g
- Fiber: 12g

3. Hormone-Balancing Sweet Potato Hash

Cook time: 15 mins / Prep time: 10 mins / Serves: 2

INGREDIENTS:

- 1 large sweet potato, peeled and diced
- 1 tbsp olive oil
- 1/2 red onion, chopped
- 1/2 bell pepper, chopped
- 1/2 tsp ground turmeric
- 1/2 tsp ground cumin
- Salt and pepper, to taste

- 2 eggs (optional for topping)

INSTRUCTIONS:

1. Heat olive oil in a large skillet over medium heat.

2. Add sweet potato and cook for about 10 minutes until softened and lightly crispy.

3. Add onion, bell pepper, turmeric, cumin, salt, and pepper. Cook for another 5 minutes.

4. Optional: Top with a fried or poached egg for added protein.

NUTRITIONAL INFORMATION (per serving):

- Calories: 290
- Protein: 8g
- Carbs: 40g
- Fat: 14g
- Fiber: 7g

4. Avocado and Egg Toast on Sprouted Bread

Cook time: 5 mins / Prep time: 5 mins / Serves: 1

INGREDIENTS:

- 1 slice sprouted grain bread
- 1/2 ripe avocado, mashed
- 1 egg (fried or poached)
- Salt and pepper, to taste
- Red pepper flakes (optional)

INSTRUCTIONS:

1. Toast the sprouted grain bread.
2. Spread the mashed avocado on top.
3. Fry or poach an egg and place it on top of the avocado.
4. Sprinkle with salt, pepper, and red pepper flakes.
5. Serve immediately.

- Calories: 300
- Protein: 12g
- Carbs: 24g
- Fat: 20g
- Fiber: 9g

5. Oatmeal with Walnuts and Cinnamon

**Cook time: 10 mins / Prep time: 5 mins / Serves: 1**

INGREDIENTS:
- 1/2 cup rolled oats and 1 cup almond milk
- 1/4 cup walnuts, chopped
- 1/2 tsp ground cinnamon
- 1 tbsp honey or maple syrup

INSTRUCTIONS:
1. In a saucepan, bring almond milk to a simmer over medium heat.
2. Add oats and cook for 5-7 minutes until soft.
3. Stir in cinnamon and sweetener of choice.
4. Top with chopped walnuts and serve.

**NUTRITIONAL INFORMATION (per serving):**
- Calories: 320
- Protein: 8g
- Carbs: 35g
- Fat: 18g
- Fiber: 6g

6. Anti-Inflammatory Golden Turmeric Latte

**Cook time: 5 mins / Prep time: 5 mins / Serves: 1**

INGREDIENTS:
- 1 cup almond milk
- 1/2 tsp ground turmeric

- 1/4 tsp black pepper
- 1 tsp honey or maple syrup
- 1/2 tsp cinnamon
- 1/4 tsp ground ginger

INSTRUCTIONS:

1. Heat almond milk in a saucepan over medium heat.
2. Stir in turmeric, black pepper, cinnamon, and ginger.
3. Simmer for 3-5 minutes, stirring occasionally.
4. Sweeten with honey or maple syrup, and serve warm.

NUTRITIONAL INFORMATION (per serving):

- Calories: 120
- Protein: 2g
- Carbs: 16g
- Fat: 7g
- Fiber: 2g

7. Greek Yogurt Parfait with Pumpkin Seeds

Cook time: 0 mins / Prep time: 5 mins / Serves: 2

INGREDIENTS:

- 1 cup Greek yogurt (unsweetened)
- 1/4 cup pumpkin seeds
- 1 tbsp chia seeds
- 1/4 cup mixed berries (blueberries, raspberries, or strawberries)
- 1 tbsp honey (optional)

INSTRUCTIONS:

1. Layer Greek yogurt, pumpkin seeds, chia seeds, and berries in a glass or bowl.
2. Drizzle with honey if desired.
3. Serve immediately or refrigerate for a few hours.

NUTRITIONAL INFORMATION (per serving):
  - Calories: 250
  - Protein: 18g
  - Carbs: 15g
  - Fat: 15g
  - Fiber: 6g

8. Banana-Almond Energy Pancakes

Cook time: 10 mins / Prep time: 5 mins / Serves: 2

INGREDIENTS:
  - 1 ripe banana, mashed
  - 2 eggs
  - 1/4 cup almond flour
  - 1/2 tsp vanilla extract
  - 1 tbsp almond butter
  - 1 tbsp maple syrup

INSTRUCTIONS:
1. In a bowl, whisk together the mashed banana, eggs, almond flour, and vanilla extract.
2. Heat a non-stick skillet over medium heat.
3. Pour batter into the skillet and cook until bubbles form on the surface (about 2-3 minutes).
4. Flip and cook for another 2-3 minutes.
5. Serve with almond butter and maple syrup.

NUTRITIONAL INFORMATION (per serving):
  - Calories: 330
  - Protein: 14g
  - Carbs: 25g
  - Fat: 22g
  - Fiber: 5g

9. Spinach and Feta Egg Muffins

Cook time: 15 mins / Prep time: 10 mins / Serves: 6 muffins

INGREDIENTS:

- 6 large eggs
- 1/2 cup spinach, chopped
- 1/4 cup feta cheese, crumbled
- Salt and pepper, to taste
- 1/4 tsp garlic powder (optional)

INSTRUCTIONS:

1. Preheat oven to 350°F (175°C).
2. In a bowl, whisk the eggs and season with salt, pepper, and garlic powder.
3. Stir in spinach and feta cheese.
4. Pour mixture into a muffin tin and bake for 12-15 minutes or until eggs are fully set.

NUTRITIONAL INFORMATION (per muffin):

- Calories: 90
- Protein: 6g
- Carbs: 2g
- Fat: 7g
- Fiber: 1g

10. Quinoa Breakfast Porridge

Cook time: 15 mins / Prep time: 5 mins / Serves: 2

INGREDIENTS:

- 1/2 cup quinoa, rinsed
- 1 cup almond milk
- 1/2 tsp ground cinnamon
- 1 tbsp chia seeds
- 1/4 cup sliced almonds
- 1 tbsp honey

<u>**INSTRUCTIONS:**</u>

1. In a saucepan, bring almond milk to a simmer.
2. Add quinoa and cook for 12-15 minutes until soft and creamy.
3. Stir in cinnamon and chia seeds.
4. Top with sliced almonds and drizzle with honey.

<u>***NUTRITIONAL INFORMATION (per serving):***</u>

- Calories: 270
- Protein: 9g
- Carbs: 38g
- Fat: 12g
- Fiber: 6g

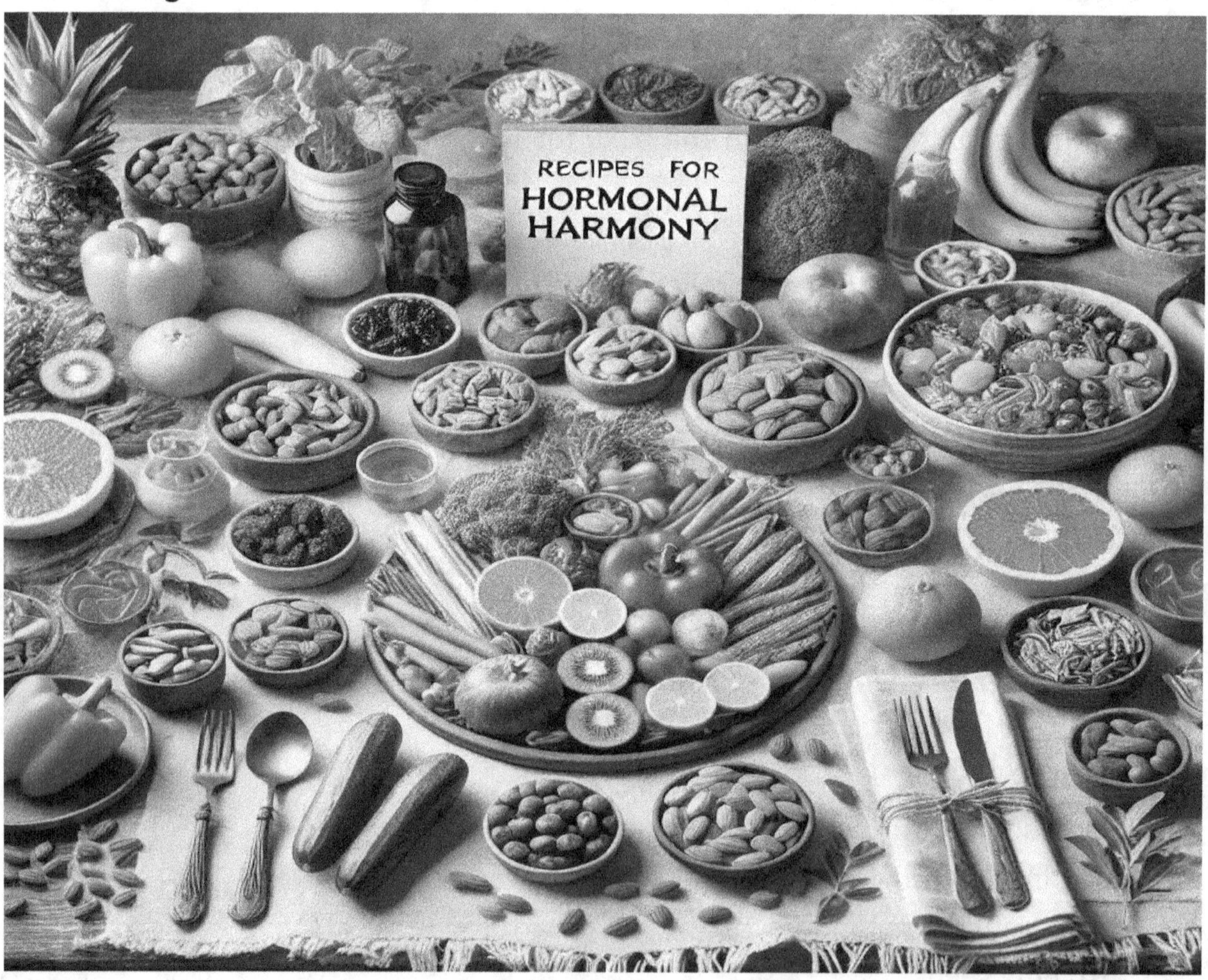

Lunch: Nutrient-Packed Midday Boosters

11. Grilled Chicken and Kale Caesar Salad

Cook time: 10 mins / Prep time: 15 mins / Serves: 2

INGREDIENTS:
- 2 chicken breasts, boneless and skinless
- 2 cups kale, chopped
- 1/4 cup Caesar dressing (use dairy-free if preferred)
- 1/4 cup grated Parmesan cheese (optional)
- 1/4 cup croutons (optional)

INSTRUCTIONS:
1. Preheat the grill to medium heat. Season chicken breasts with salt, pepper, and a drizzle of olive oil. Grill for 6-7 minutes per side until cooked through.
2. Slice the grilled chicken into strips.
3. In a large bowl, toss chopped kale with Caesar dressing until well coated.
4. Top with grilled chicken, Parmesan cheese, and croutons. Serve immediately.

NUTRITIONAL INFORMATION (per serving):
- Calories: 350
- Protein: 40g
- Carbs: 15g
- Fat: 18g
- Fiber: 5g

12. Wild-Caught Salmon Power Bowl

Cook time: 10 mins / Prep time: 10 mins / Serves: 2

INGREDIENTS:
- 2 wild-caught salmon fillets
- 1 cup quinoa, cooked
- 1/2 avocado, sliced
- 1/4 cup cucumber, sliced

- 1/4 cup shredded carrots
- 1 tbsp olive oil
- 1 tbsp lemon juice
- Salt and pepper, to taste

INSTRUCTIONS:

1. Preheat the oven to 400°F (200°C). Place salmon fillets on a baking sheet lined with parchment paper. Drizzle with olive oil, lemon juice, and season with salt and pepper.
2. Bake for 10-12 minutes, or until salmon flakes easily with a fork.
3. Assemble bowls by layering cooked quinoa, avocado slices, cucumber, and shredded carrots.
4. Top with baked salmon and serve immediately.

NUTRITIONAL INFORMATION (per serving):

- Calories: 420
- Protein: 35g
- Carbs: 30g
- Fat: 25g
- Fiber: 9g

13. Turkey and Avocado Lettuce Wraps

Cook time: 5 mins / Prep time: 5 mins / Serves: 2

INGREDIENTS:

- 1 lb ground turkey
- 1 avocado, sliced
- 1 head of Romaine lettuce, leaves separated
- 1/4 cup red onion, thinly sliced
- 1 tbsp olive oil
- Salt and pepper, to taste
- 1 tsp chili powder (optional)

<u>**INSTRUCTIONS:**</u>

1. In a skillet, heat olive oil over medium heat. Add ground turkey, season with salt, pepper, and chili powder. Cook until browned, about 5-7 minutes.
2. Spoon turkey mixture onto Romaine lettuce leaves.
3. Top with avocado slices and red onion.
4. Wrap up the lettuce and serve.

<u>***NUTRITIONAL INFORMATION (per serving):***</u>
  - Calories: 350
  - Protein: 30g
  - Carbs: 15g
  - Fat: 22g
  - Fiber: 7g

14. Lentil and Sweet Potato Stew

Cook time: 30 mins / Prep time: 10 mins / Serves: 4

<u>**INGREDIENTS:**</u>
  - 1 cup green lentils, rinsed
  - 2 large sweet potatoes, peeled and diced
  - 1 onion, chopped
  - 2 cloves garlic, minced
  - 1 can diced tomatoes (14 oz)
  - 4 cups vegetable broth
  - 1 tsp cumin
  - 1 tsp turmeric
  - Salt and pepper, to taste
  - 2 tbsp olive oil

<u>**INSTRUCTIONS:**</u>

1. In a large pot, heat olive oil over medium heat. Add onion and garlic, sauté for 2-3 minutes.
2. Add diced sweet potatoes, cumin, turmeric, and salt. Stir to coat.
3. Add lentils, diced tomatoes, and vegetable broth. Bring to a simmer, cover, and cook for 25-30 minutes, until lentils and sweet potatoes are tender.

4. Adjust seasoning with salt and pepper, and serve.

NUTRITIONAL INFORMATION (per serving):
   - Calories: 280
   - Protein: 12g
   - Carbs: 50g
   - Fat: 7g
   - Fiber: 14g

15. Detox Buddha Bowl with Tahini Dressing

Cook time: 10 mins / Prep time: 15 mins / Serves: 2

INGREDIENTS:
   - 1 cup cooked brown rice
   - 1/2 cup chickpeas, cooked
   - 1/2 cup steamed broccoli
   - 1/2 avocado, sliced
   - 1/4 cup shredded carrots
   - 2 tbsp tahini
   - 1 tbsp lemon juice
   - 1 tsp maple syrup
   - Salt and pepper, to taste

INSTRUCTIONS:
1. Assemble the bowl by layering brown rice, chickpeas, steamed broccoli, avocado slices, and shredded carrots.
2. In a small bowl, whisk together tahini, lemon juice, maple syrup, salt, and pepper.
3. Drizzle tahini dressing over the Buddha bowl and serve.

NUTRITIONAL INFORMATION (per serving):
   - Calories: 380
   - Protein: 15g
   - Carbs: 50g
   - Fat: 17g

- Fiber: 14g

16. Hormone-Friendly Veggie Stir-Fry

Cook time: 15 mins / Prep time: 10 mins / Serves: 2

INGREDIENTS:
- 1 cup broccoli florets
- 1/2 cup red bell pepper, sliced
- 1/2 cup snow peas
- 1/4 cup carrots, julienne and 2 tbsp coconut oil
- 1 tbsp soy sauce or coconut aminos
- 1 tsp sesame oil
- 1 tbsp sesame seeds
- 1 tbsp fresh cilantro, chopped

INSTRUCTIONS:
1. Heat coconut oil in a skillet over medium heat. Add broccoli, bell pepper, snow peas, and carrots. Stir-fry for 5-7 minutes until vegetables are tender.
2. Stir in soy sauce, sesame oil, and sesame seeds. Cook for another 1-2 minutes.
3. Garnish with fresh cilantro and serve.

NUTRITIONAL INFORMATION (per serving):
- Calories: 250
- Protein: 6g
- Carbs: 30g
- Fat: 14g
- Fiber: 8g

17. Chickpea and Quinoa Salad

Cook time: 15 mins / Prep time: 5 mins / Serves: 2

INGREDIENTS:
- 1 cup cooked quinoa
- 1 can chickpeas (14 oz), drained and rinsed
- 1/2 cucumber, diced

- 1/2 red onion, diced
- 1/4 cup fresh parsley, chopped
- 2 tbsp olive oil
- 1 tbsp lemon juice
- Salt and pepper, to taste

INSTRUCTIONS:

1. In a large bowl, combine quinoa, chickpeas, cucumber, red onion, and parsley.
2. Drizzle with olive oil and lemon juice.
3. Toss to combine and season with salt and pepper.
4. Serve chilled or at room temperature.

NUTRITIONAL INFORMATION (per serving):

- Calories: 350
- Protein: 12g
- Carbs: 45g
- Fat: 14g
- Fiber: 10g

18. Spinach and Mushroom Frittata

Cook time: 20 mins / Prep time: 10 mins / Serves: 4

INGREDIENTS:

- 6 large eggs
- 1 cup spinach, chopped
- 1/2 cup mushrooms, sliced
- 1/4 cup feta cheese, crumbled
- 1/4 cup milk
- 1 tbsp olive oil
- Salt and pepper, to taste

INSTRUCTIONS:

1. Preheat oven to 350°F (175°C).
2. In an oven-safe skillet, heat olive oil over medium heat. Sauté mushrooms and spinach until softened.

3. In a bowl, whisk eggs with milk, salt, and pepper. Pour over the vegetables in the skillet.

4. Sprinkle feta cheese on top and bake for 15-20 minutes until set.

NUTRITIONAL INFORMATION (per serving):
- Calories: 250
- Protein: 18g
- Carbs: 5g
- Fat: 18g
- Fiber: 2g

19. Mediterranean Tuna Salad with Olives

Cook time: 5 mins / Prep time: 5 mins / Serves: 2

INGREDIENTS:
- 1 can tuna in olive oil (drained)
- 1/4 cup Kalamata olives, pitted and sliced
- 1/2 cucumber, diced
- 1/4 red onion, diced
- 1 tbsp capers
- 2 tbsp olive oil
- 1 tbsp lemon juice
- Salt and pepper, to taste

INSTRUCTIONS:
1. In a bowl, combine tuna, olives, cucumber, onion, and capers.
2. Drizzle with olive oil and lemon juice.
3. Toss to combine and season with salt and pepper.

NUTRITIONAL INFORMATION (per serving):
- Calories: 320
- Protein: 25g
- Carbs: 5g
- Fat: 22g
- Fiber: 2g

20. Curried Cauliflower and Rice Bowl

Cook time: 15 mins / Prep time: 5 mins / Serves: 2

INGREDIENTS:

- 1 head cauliflower, broken into florets
- 1 cup cooked brown rice
- 1 tbsp coconut oil
- 1 tsp curry powder
- Salt and pepper, to taste
- 1/4 cup chopped cilantro
- 1 tbsp sesame seeds (optional)

INSTRUCTIONS:

1. Preheat oven to 400°F (200°C).

2. Toss cauliflower florets with coconut oil, curry powder, salt, and pepper. Roast for 15-20 minutes.

3. Assemble bowls by layering rice, roasted cauliflower, and sprinkling with cilantro and sesame seeds.

NUTRITIONAL INFORMATION (per serving):

- Calories: 320
- Protein: 8g
- Carbs: 45g
- Fat: 14g
- Fiber: 9g

Dinner: Soothing Evening Dishes

21. Lemon Herb Baked Salmon with Asparagus

Cook time: 20 mins / Prep time: 5 mins / Serves: 2

INGREDIENTS:

- 2 salmon fillets
- 1 bunch asparagus, trimmed
- 1 tbsp olive oil and 1 tbsp lemon juice
- 1 tsp dried thyme and 1 tsp garlic powder
- Salt and pepper, to taste
- Lemon slices, for garnish

INSTRUCTIONS:

1. Preheat the oven to 375°F (190°C).
2. Place salmon fillets on a baking sheet lined with parchment paper. Drizzle with olive oil and lemon juice, then sprinkle with thyme, garlic powder, salt, and pepper.
3. Arrange asparagus around the salmon and drizzle with olive oil.
4. Bake for 15-18 minutes until the salmon flakes easily with a fork.
5. Garnish with lemon slices and serve.

NUTRITIONAL INFORMATION (per serving):

- Calories: 370
- Protein: 32g
- Carbs: 10g
- Fat: 24g
- Fiber: 5g

22. Garlic-Roasted Chicken with Root Vegetables

Cook time: 40 mins / Prep time: 10 mins / Serves: 4

INGREDIENTS:

- 4 bone-in, skin-on chicken thighs
- 2 carrots, peeled and chopped

- 2 parsnips, peeled and chopped
- 1 sweet potato, peeled and cubed
- 3 tbsp olive oil
- 4 cloves garlic, minced
- 1 tbsp rosemary, chopped
- Salt and pepper, to taste

INSTRUCTIONS:

1. Preheat the oven to 400°F (200°C).

2. In a large bowl, toss chopped vegetables with 1 tablespoon of olive oil, rosemary, salt, and pepper.

3. Arrange chicken thighs on a baking sheet and rub with olive oil, minced garlic, salt, and pepper.

4. Scatter vegetables around the chicken.

5. Roast for 35-40 minutes, until chicken is cooked through and vegetables are tender.

NUTRITIONAL INFORMATION (per serving):

- Calories: 430
- Protein: 35g
- Carbs: 30g
- Fat: 22g
- Fiber: 8g

23. Coconut Curry Shrimp with Zucchini Noodles

Cook time: 15 mins / Prep time: 10 mins / Serves: 2

INGREDIENTS:

- 1 lb shrimp, peeled and deveined
- 2 zucchinis, spiralized into noodles
- 1 can (13 oz) coconut milk
- 2 tbsp curry powder
- 1 tbsp olive oil
- 1/2 onion, chopped
- 2 cloves garlic, minced

- Salt and pepper, to taste
- Fresh cilantro, for garnish

INSTRUCTIONS:

1. In a skillet, heat olive oil over medium heat. Add onions and garlic, sauté until softened (about 3 minutes).

2. Add shrimp and cook for 2-3 minutes until pink.

3. Stir in coconut milk and curry powder. Let it simmer for 3-4 minutes.

4. In another pan, sauté zucchini noodles for 2-3 minutes until tender.

5. Serve the shrimp and curry sauce over the zucchini noodles, garnished with fresh cilantro.

__NUTRITIONAL INFORMATION (per serving)__:

- Calories: 360
- Protein: 30g
- Carbs: 15g
- Fat: 22g
- Fiber: 4g

24. Stuffed Bell Peppers with Ground Turkey

Cook time: 30 mins / Prep time: 10 mins / Serves: 4

INGREDIENTS:

- 4 bell peppers, tops cut off and seeds removed
- 1 lb ground turkey
- 1/2 cup cooked quinoa
- 1 can diced tomatoes (14 oz)
- 1 tbsp olive oil
- 1/2 onion, chopped
- 1 tsp cumin
- 1 tsp paprika
- Salt and pepper, to taste
- 1/4 cup shredded cheese (optional)

<u>**INSTRUCTIONS:**</u>

1. Preheat the oven to 375°F (190°C).

2. Heat olive oil in a skillet over medium heat. Add chopped onion and sauté for 3 minutes.

3. Add ground turkey, cumin, paprika, salt, and pepper. Cook until browned, about 7-8 minutes.

4. Stir in diced tomatoes and cooked quinoa.

5. Stuff the bell peppers with the turkey mixture and place them in a baking dish.

6. Bake for 20 minutes, topping with cheese (if using) in the last 5 minutes.

<u>***NUTRITIONAL INFORMATION (per serving):***</u>

- Calories: 330
- Protein: 30g
- Carbs: 20g
- Fat: 15g
- Fiber: 6g

25. Hormone-Boosting Beef and Broccoli Stir-Fry

Cook time: 20 mins / Prep time: 10 mins / Serves: 2

<u>**INGREDIENTS:**</u>

- 1 lb grass-fed beef, thinly sliced
- 2 cups broccoli florets
- 2 tbsp olive oil
- 2 tbsp coconut aminos (or soy sauce)
- 2 tbsp sesame oil
- 2 cloves garlic, minced
- 1 tsp ginger, grated
- 1 tbsp sesame seeds, for garnish

<u>**INSTRUCTIONS:**</u>

1. Heat olive oil in a large skillet or wok over medium-high heat. Add beef and stir-fry for 3-4 minutes, until browned.

2. Add garlic, ginger, and broccoli florets. Stir-fry for 4-5 minutes until broccoli is tender but still crisp.

3. Stir in coconut aminos and sesame oil. Cook for 1-2 more minutes.

4. Garnish with sesame seeds and serve.

NUTRITIONAL INFORMATION (per serving):
- Calories: 380
- Protein: 40g
- Carbs: 15g
- Fat: 22g
- Fiber: 6g

26. Grilled Halibut with Quinoa Pilaf

Cook time: 15 mins / Prep time: 10 mins / Serves: 2

INGREDIENTS:
- 2 halibut fillets
- 1 cup quinoa, cooked
- 1 tbsp olive oil
- 1 tbsp lemon juice
- 1/4 cup parsley, chopped
- Salt and pepper, to taste
- 1/2 cup cucumber, diced

INSTRUCTIONS:
1. Preheat the grill to medium-high heat. Drizzle halibut fillets with olive oil and season with salt and pepper.

2. Grill halibut for 3-4 minutes per side until cooked through.

3. In a separate bowl, mix cooked quinoa with cucumber, parsley, lemon juice, salt, and pepper.

4. Serve halibut fillets on top of quinoa pilaf.

NUTRITIONAL INFORMATION (per serving):
- Calories: 330
- Protein: 35g
- Carbs: 25g
- Fat: 12g

- Fiber: 5g

27. Spinach and Ricotta Stuffed Portobello Mushrooms
Cook time: 25 mins / Prep time: 10 mins / Serves: 2

INGREDIENTS:
- 4 large Portobello mushrooms, stems removed
- 1 cup spinach, chopped
- 1/2 cup ricotta cheese
- 1/4 cup grated Parmesan cheese and 2 tbsp olive oil
- 1 clove garlic, minced
- Salt and pepper, to taste

INSTRUCTIONS:
1. Preheat the oven to 375°F (190°C).
2. Sauté garlic and spinach in olive oil for 2-3 minutes until wilted.
3. In a bowl, mix spinach with ricotta and Parmesan. Season with salt and pepper.
4. Stuff mushrooms with the spinach-ricotta mixture and place them on a baking sheet.
5. Bake for 20-25 minutes until mushrooms are tender.

NUTRITIONAL INFORMATION (per serving):
- Calories: 260
- Protein: 16g
- Carbs: 14g
- Fat: 18g
- Fiber: 6g

28. Zesty Citrus Baked Cod with Steamed Greens
Cook time: 20 mins / Prep time: 5 mins / Serves: 2

INGREDIENTS:
- 2 cod fillets
- 1 tbsp olive oil
- Juice of 1 orange

- Zest of 1 lemon
- 1 tsp paprika
- Salt and pepper, to taste
- 2 cups mixed greens (spinach, kale, arugula), steamed

INSTRUCTIONS:

1. Preheat the oven to 375°F (190°C).

2. Place cod fillets on a baking sheet, drizzle with olive oil, orange juice, and season with paprika, salt, and pepper.

3. Bake for 15-18 minutes until the fish flakes easily.

4. Serve the cod over a bed of steamed greens.

NUTRITIONAL INFORMATION (per serving):

- Calories: 280
- Protein: 28g
- Carbs: 10g
- Fat: 14g
- Fiber: 4g

29. Lentil and Mushroom Shepherd's Pie

Cook time: 40 mins / Prep time: 15 mins / Serves: 4

INGREDIENTS:

- 1 cup lentils, cooked
- 1 cup mushrooms, chopped and 1/2 onion, chopped
- 2 cloves garlic, minced
- 1 cup vegetable broth and 1 tbsp olive oil
- 2 large potatoes, peeled and mashed
- Salt and pepper, to taste

INSTRUCTIONS:

1. Preheat the oven to 375°F (190°C).

2. In a skillet, heat olive oil and sauté onion, garlic, and mushrooms for 5 minutes.

3. Stir in cooked lentils and vegetable broth. Cook for 10-15 minutes, reducing the broth.

4. Place lentil-mushroom mixture in a baking dish, and top with mashed potatoes.

5. Bake for 20-25 minutes until golden on top.

NUTRITIONAL INFORMATION (per serving):
   - Calories: 350
   - Protein: 20g
   - Carbs: 45g
   - Fat: 12g
   - Fiber: 9g

30. Warm Chicken and Sweet Potato Bowl

Cook time: 30 mins / Prep time: 10 mins / Serves: 2

INGREDIENTS:
   - 2 chicken breasts
   - 2 sweet potatoes, peeled and cubed
   - 1 tbsp olive oil and 1 tsp paprika
   - Salt and pepper, to taste
   - 1/2 cup spinach, wilted

INSTRUCTIONS:
1. Preheat the oven to 400°F (200°C).

2. Toss sweet potatoes with olive oil, paprika, salt, and pepper. Roast for 25 minutes.

3. Season chicken breasts with salt and pepper, and cook in a skillet for 6-8 minutes per side until cooked through.

4. Assemble bowls by layering roasted sweet potatoes, spinach, and sliced chicken.

NUTRITIONAL INFORMATION (per serving):
   - Calories: 380
   - Protein: 35g
   - Carbs: 40g
   - Fat: 12g
   - Fiber: 7g

31. Anti-Stress Matcha Energy Balls

Cook time: 10 mins / Prep time: 5 mins / Makes: 12 balls

INGREDIENTS:
  - 1 cup rolled oats
  - 2 tbsp matcha powder
  - 1/4 cup almond butter
  - 1 tbsp honey
  - 1/4 cup unsweetened shredded coconut
  - 1 tbsp chia seeds
  - 1 tsp vanilla extract

INSTRUCTIONS:
1. In a bowl, combine all ingredients and mix until well combined.
2. Roll the mixture into small balls, about 1 inch in diameter.
3. Chill in the fridge for at least 30 minutes before serving.

NUTRITIONAL INFORMATION (per serving):
  - Calories: 140
  - Protein: 4g
  - Carbs: 18g
  - Fat: 7g
  - Fiber: 3g

32. Apple Slices with Almond Butter

Cook time: 5 mins / Prep time: 5 mins / Serves: 2

INGREDIENTS:
  - 2 apples, sliced
  - 1/4 cup almond butter
  - Cinnamon, for sprinkling (optional)

INSTRUCTIONS:

1. Slice the apples into wedges.

2. Serve with almond butter on the side for dipping, and sprinkle with cinnamon if desired.

NUTRITIONAL INFORMATION (per serving):

   - Calories: 250
   - Protein: 4g
   - Carbs: 30g
   - Fat: 15g
   - Fiber: 6g

33. Berry-Collagen Smoothie

Cook time: 5 mins / Prep time: 5 mins / Serves: 1

INGREDIENTS:

   - 1/2 cup mixed berries (strawberries, blueberries, raspberries)
   - 1 scoop collagen powder
   - 1/2 cup unsweetened almond milk
   - 1/2 banana
   - 1 tsp honey (optional)

INSTRUCTIONS:

1. Blend all ingredients until smooth.

2. Pour into a glass and enjoy immediately.

NUTRITIONAL INFORMATION (per serving):

   - Calories: 180
   - Protein: 15g
   - Carbs: 20g
   - Fat: 5g
   - Fiber: 5g

34. Homemade Trail Mix with Dark Chocolate

Cook time: 5 mins / Prep time: 5 mins / Serves: 4

INGREDIENTS:
- 1/2 cup almonds
- 1/2 cup cashews
- 1/4 cup pumpkin seeds
- 1/4 cup dark chocolate chips (70% cocoa)
- 1/4 cup dried cranberries

INSTRUCTIONS:
1. Combine all ingredients in a bowl.
2. Toss to mix evenly and serve in portions.

NUTRITIONAL INFORMATION (per serving):
- Calories: 200
- Protein: 5g
- Carbs: 18g
- Fat: 14g
- Fiber: 4g

35. Roasted Chickpeas with Paprika

Cook time: 30 mins / Prep time: 5 mins / Serves: 4

INGREDIENTS:
- 1 can chickpeas, drained and rinsed
- 1 tbsp olive oil
- 1 tsp paprika
- 1/2 tsp garlic powder
- Salt, to taste

INSTRUCTIONS:
1. Preheat the oven to 400°F (200°C).
2. Toss chickpeas with olive oil, paprika, garlic powder, and salt.

3. Spread chickpeas on a baking sheet and roast for 25-30 minutes, shaking the pan halfway through.

4. Let cool before serving.

NUTRITIONAL INFORMATION (per serving):
- Calories: 150
- Protein: 7g
- Carbs: 20g
- Fat: 7g
- Fiber: 6g

36. Hormone-Balancing Green Juice

Cook time: 5 mins / Prep time: 5 mins / Serves: 1

INGREDIENTS:
- 1 cucumber, chopped
- 1 cup spinach
- 1/2 lemon, juiced
- 1-inch piece ginger, peeled
- 1 green apple, chopped
- 1/2 cup water or coconut water

INSTRUCTIONS:
1. Blend all ingredients together until smooth.
2. Strain through a fine mesh if you prefer a smoother juice.

NUTRITIONAL INFORMATION (per serving):
- Calories: 70
- Protein: 2g
- Carbs: 16g
- Fat: 0g
- Fiber: 4g

37. Turmeric-Honey Roasted Almonds

Cook time: 20 mins / Prep time: 5 mins / Serves: 4

INGREDIENTS:

- 1 cup raw almonds
- 1 tbsp olive oil
- 1/2 tsp turmeric
- 1 tbsp honey
- 1/4 tsp cinnamon
- Salt, to taste

INSTRUCTIONS:

1. Preheat the oven to 350°F (175°C).
2. Toss almonds with olive oil, turmeric, honey, cinnamon, and salt.
3. Spread almonds on a baking sheet and roast for 15-20 minutes, stirring halfway through.
4. Let cool before serving.

NUTRITIONAL INFORMATION (per serving):

- Calories: 180
- Protein: 6g
- Carbs: 9g
- Fat: 15g
- Fiber: 3g

38. Avocado-Lime Dip with Veggie Sticks

Cook time: 5 mins / Prep time: 5 mins / Serves: 2

INGREDIENTS:

- 1 ripe avocado
- Juice of 1 lime
- 1 tbsp olive oil
- Salt and pepper, to taste
- Veggie sticks (carrots, celery, cucumber, bell peppers)

INSTRUCTIONS:

1. Mash the avocado in a bowl.

2. Stir in lime juice, olive oil, salt, and pepper until smooth.

3. Serve with veggie sticks for dipping.

NUTRITIONAL INFORMATION (per serving):

- Calories: 220
- Protein: 3g
- Carbs: 16g
- Fat: 18g
- Fiber: 10g

39. Coconut Bliss Balls with Chia Seeds

Cook time: 10 mins / Prep time: 5 mins / Makes: 12 balls

INGREDIENTS:

- 1 cup unsweetened shredded coconut
- 1/4 cup chia seeds
- 1/4 cup almond butter
- 1 tbsp honey
- 1 tsp vanilla extract

INSTRUCTIONS:

1. In a bowl, mix all ingredients until well combined.

2. Roll the mixture into small balls.

3. Chill in the fridge for 30 minutes before serving.

NUTRITIONAL INFORMATION (per serving):

- Calories: 160
- Protein: 4g
- Carbs: 14g
- Fat: 12g
- Fiber: 6g

Cook time: 5 mins / Prep time: 5 mins / Serves: 4

INGREDIENTS:

- 2 cups plain Greek yogurt
- 1/2 cup blueberries
- 1 tbsp honey
- 1/4 tsp vanilla extract
- 2 tbsp chopped almonds

INSTRUCTIONS:

1. Spread yogurt onto a parchment-lined baking sheet.
2. Drizzle with honey and vanilla, then sprinkle with blueberries and chopped almonds.
3. Freeze for 2-3 hours until firm.
4. Break into pieces and serve.

NUTRITIONAL INFORMATION (per serving):

- Calories: 120
- Protein: 8g
- Carbs: 14g
- Fat: 5g
- Fiber: 3g

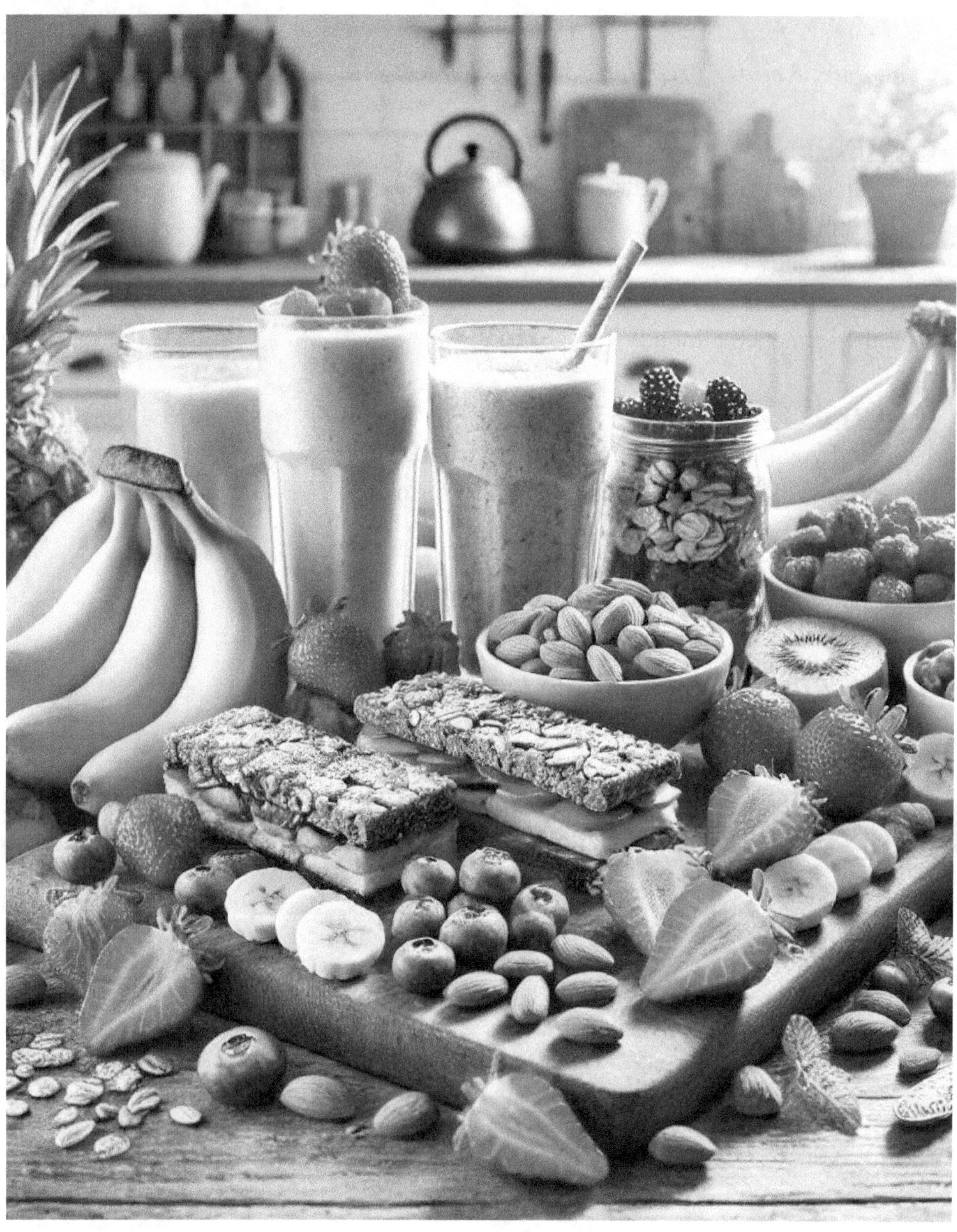

21-Day Meal Plan for the Cortisol Detox Diet Plan

This 21-day meal plan is tailored to help you lower cortisol levels, balance your hormones, and nourish your body. Each day features breakfast, lunch, dinner, and one snack to keep it simple yet effective. Recipes are packed with nutrient-dense, stress-relieving ingredients.

<u>Week 1</u>

Day 1
  - **Breakfast:** <u>Stress-Busting Green Smoothie Bowl</u>
  - **Snack:** <u>Apple Slices with Almond Butter</u>
  - **Lunch:** <u>Grilled Chicken and Kale Caesar Salad</u>
  - **Dinner:** <u>Lemon Herb Baked Salmon with Asparagus</u>

Day 2
  - **Breakfast:** <u>Oatmeal with Walnuts and Cinnamon</u>
  - **Snack:** <u>Anti-Stress Matcha Energy Balls</u>
  - **Lunch:** <u>Chickpea and Quinoa Salad</u>
  - **Dinner:** <u>Coconut Curry Shrimp with Zucchini Noodles</u>

Day 3
  - **Breakfast:** <u>Avocado and Egg Toast on Sprouted Bread</u>
  - **Snack:** <u>Turmeric-Honey Roasted Almonds</u>
  - **Lunch:** <u>Lentil and Sweet Potato Stew</u>
  - **Dinner:** <u>Stuffed Bell Peppers with Ground Turkey</u>

Day 4
  - **Breakfast:** <u>Spinach and Feta Egg Muffins</u>
  - **Snack:** <u>Hormone-Balancing Green Juice</u>
  - **Lunch:** <u>Mediterranean Tuna Salad with Olives</u>
  - **Dinner:** <u>Hormone-Boosting Beef and Broccoli Stir-Fry</u>

Day 5
  - **Breakfast:** <u>Greek Yogurt Parfait with Pumpkin Seeds</u>

- **Snack:** Berry-Collagen Smoothie
- **Lunch:** Spinach and Mushroom Frittata
- **Dinner:** Garlic-Roasted Chicken with Root Vegetables

Day 6
- **Breakfast:** Quinoa Breakfast Porridge
- **Snack:** Homemade Trail Mix with Dark Chocolate
- **Lunch:** Detox Buddha Bowl with Tahini Dressing
- **Dinner:** Zesty Citrus Baked Cod with Steamed Greens

Day 7
- **Breakfast:** Banana-Almond Energy Pancakes
- **Snack:** Roasted Chickpeas with Paprika
- **Lunch:** Wild-Caught Salmon Power Bowl
- **Dinner:** Warm Chicken and Sweet Potato Bowl

Week 2

Day 8
- **Breakfast:** Sweet Potato Hash with Avocado
- **Snack:** Coconut Bliss Balls with Chia Seeds
- **Lunch:** Turkey and Avocado Lettuce Wraps
- **Dinner:** Grilled Halibut with Quinoa Pilaf

Day 9
- **Breakfast:** Overnight Chia Pudding with Berries
- **Snack:** Hormone-Friendly Veggie Sticks with Avocado Dip
- **Lunch:** Lentil and Mushroom Shepherd's Pie
- **Dinner:** Spinach and Ricotta Stuffed Portobello Mushrooms

Day 10
- **Breakfast:** Hormone-Balancing Sweet Potato Hash
- **Snack:** Roasted Chickpeas with Paprika
- **Lunch:** Detox Buddha Bowl with Tahini Dressing
- **Dinner:** Garlic-Roasted Chicken with Root Vegetables

Day 11
   - **Breakfast:** Stress-Busting Green Smoothie Bowl
   - **Snack:** Hormone-Balancing Green Juice
   - **Lunch:** Mediterranean Tuna Salad with Olives
   - **Dinner:** Coconut Curry Shrimp with Zucchini Noodles

Day 12
   - **Breakfast:** Spinach and Feta Egg Muffins
   - **Snack:** Anti-Stress Matcha Energy Balls
   - **Lunch:** Wild-Caught Salmon Power Bowl
   - **Dinner:** Zesty Citrus Baked Cod with Steamed Greens

Day 13
   - **Breakfast:** Banana-Almond Energy Pancakes
   - **Snack:** Berry-Collagen Smoothie
   - **Lunch:** Grilled Chicken and Kale Caesar Salad
   - **Dinner:** Hormone-Boosting Beef and Broccoli Stir-Fry

Day 14
   - **Breakfast:** Greek Yogurt Parfait with Pumpkin Seeds
   - **Snack:** Turmeric-Honey Roasted Almonds
   - **Lunch:** Chickpea and Quinoa Salad
   - **Dinner:** Lentil and Sweet Potato Stew

Week 3
Day 15
   - **Breakfast:** Quinoa Breakfast Porridge
   - **Snack:** Coconut Bliss Balls with Chia Seeds
   - **Lunch:** Spinach and Mushroom Frittata
   - **Dinner:** Warm Chicken and Sweet Potato Bowl

Day 16
   - **Breakfast:** Avocado and Egg Toast on Sprouted Bread
   - **Snack:** Apple Slices with Almond Butter
   - **Lunch:** Turkey and Avocado Lettuce Wraps

- **Dinner:** <u>Lemon Herb Baked Salmon with Asparagus</u>

Day 17
   - **Breakfast:** <u>Sweet Potato Hash with Avocado</u>
   - **Snack:** <u>Homemade Trail Mix with Dark Chocolate</u>
   - **Lunch:** <u>Lentil and Mushroom Shepherd's Pie</u>
   - **Dinner:** <u>Grilled Halibut with Quinoa Pilaf</u>

Day 18
   - **Breakfast:** <u>Stress-Busting Green Smoothie Bowl</u>
   - **Snack:** <u>Hormone-Balancing Green Juice</u>
   - **Lunch:** <u>Wild-Caught Salmon Power Bowl</u>
   - **Dinner:** <u>Stuffed Bell Peppers with Ground Turkey</u>

Day 19
   - **Breakfast:** <u>Banana-Almond Energy Pancakes</u>
   - **Snack:** <u>Roasted Chickpeas with Paprika</u>
   - **Lunch:** <u>Mediterranean Tuna Salad with Olives</u>
   - **Dinner:** <u>Spinach and Ricotta Stuffed Portobello Mushrooms</u>

Day 20
   - **Breakfast:** <u>Oatmeal with Walnuts and Cinnamon</u>
   - **Snack:** <u>Turmeric-Honey Roasted Almonds</u>
   - **Lunch:** <u>Grilled Chicken and Kale Caesar Salad</u>
   - **Dinner:** <u>Garlic-Roasted Chicken with Root Vegetables</u>

Day 21
   - **Breakfast:** <u>Overnight Chia Pudding with Berries</u>
   - **Snack:** <u>Berry-Collagen Smoothie</u>
   - **Lunch:** <u>Detox Buddha Bowl with Tahini Dressing</u>
   - **Dinner:** <u>Coconut Curry Shrimp with Zucchini Noodles</u>

This meal plan provides a balance of nutrients to support cortisol detox and promote overall wellness. Adjust portion sizes and repeat favorite meals as needed to suit your preferences.

CONCLUSION

Your Path to Sustainable Health

Achieving hormonal balance and managing cortisol levels is not a one-time event, but rather a lifelong commitment to taking care of your body and mind. By integrating the principles of the Cortisol Detox Diet Plan into your daily routine, you are setting yourself on a path to not only manage stress and improve hormonal health but also to create lasting habits that will support your overall well-being.

Remember, this journey isn't about perfection; it's about progress. There will be days when you feel like you're on top of the world and days when challenges arise. What matters most is the dedication to continually strive for better health, to listen to your body, and to nurture it in ways that enhance your energy, mood, and vitality.

Each day, as you follow the guidelines provided in this book—whether through meals, stress management, or lifestyle changes—you will move closer to a balanced, healthy life. The path you've chosen is one of empowerment, and as you transform your health, you also begin to transform your life. You are building a foundation that supports not just your body, but your mind and spirit as well.

Tips for Staying on Track

Staying committed to the principles of this detox program requires both planning and consistency. Here are a few tips to ensure long-term success:

1. Plan Ahead: Meal prepping is key to success: Take time each week to prepare your meals, snacks, and grocery list. This will save you time and prevent unhealthy choices when hunger strikes.

2. Stay Hydrated: Drinking plenty of water is essential for detoxification and overall well-being. Keep a water bottle with you and aim to drink at least 8 cups a day.

3. Practice Mindfulness: Integrate short moments of mindfulness throughout your day, whether through deep breathing, a quick meditation, or simply taking a moment to relax. This helps reduce stress and keeps cortisol levels in check.

4. Be Kind to Yourself: Remember, health is a journey. Celebrate your successes, no matter how small, and forgive yourself for the occasional slip-up. This process is about progress, not perfection.

5. Continue Learning: Stay informed about how stress affects your health and explore new ways to manage it. This will keep you motivated and help you build a lifestyle of balance.

6. Build Support: Share your journey with a friend, family member, or support group. Having accountability partners can make the process easier and more enjoyable.

By integrating these tips into your life, you'll set yourself up for sustainable health and lasting hormonal balance. This is just the beginning of a new chapter for your well-being. Stay committed, trust the process, and enjoy the transformation as you continue your journey to hormonal harmony. Your body will thank you.

BONUS

Shopping List for Cortisol Detox Success

To ensure your Cortisol Detox Diet Plan is as effective as possible, having the right ingredients on hand is crucial. Below is a comprehensive shopping list of foods that will support your detox and hormonal balance. Feel free to customize it based on your preferences and dietary needs.

Proteins:
- Wild-caught salmon
- Chicken breast or thighs (preferably organic, free-range)
- Grass-fed beef
- Turkey breast
- Organic eggs
- Tofu or tempeh (for plant-based options)
- Canned tuna (in water or olive oil)

Vegetables:
- Kale, spinach, and Swiss chard
- Broccoli, cauliflower, and Brussels sprouts
- Sweet potatoes and yams
- Zucchini, squash, and cucumber
- Bell peppers, tomatoes, and carrots
- Mushrooms (shiitake, portobello, or button)
- Asparagus, green beans, and snap peas
- Avocados
- Garlic and onions

Fruits:
- Blueberries, strawberries, and raspberries
- Apples, pears, and bananas
- Oranges, lemons, and grapefruits
- Pomegranates and kiwi
- Coconut (fresh or dried)

Whole Grains & Legumes:
- Quinoa, brown rice, and wild rice
- Oats (steel-cut or rolled)
- Lentils, chickpeas, and black beans
- Chia seeds, hemp seeds, and flaxseeds

Nuts & Seeds:
- Almonds, walnuts, and cashews
- Pumpkin seeds and sunflower seeds
- Chia seeds and flaxseeds
- Nut butters (almond, peanut, or sunflower butter)

Healthy Fats:
- Extra virgin olive oil
- Coconut oil
- Avocado oil
- Ghee (clarified butter)

Dairy & Dairy Alternatives:
- Greek yogurt (plain, unsweetened)
- Almond milk, coconut milk, or oat milk (unsweetened)
- Unsweetened coconut yogurt

Herbs, Spices & Seasonings:
- Fresh ginger, turmeric, and cilantro
- Cinnamon, cumin, and paprika
- Sea salt and black pepper
- Apple cider vinegar
- Tamari (gluten-free soy sauce)
- Fresh herbs like basil, parsley, and thyme

Beverages:
- Green tea (matcha or regular)
- Herbal teas (peppermint, chamomile, or ginger)

- Freshly squeezed lemon juice
- Coconut water

Supplements and Tools to Support Your Journey

While food is the foundation of this detox program, supplements and tools can offer additional support for managing cortisol levels and improving overall health. Here's a guide to the best supplements and tools that can enhance your detox experience:

<u>Supplements:</u>

1. Ashwagandha: An adaptogen herb known for its ability to lower cortisol and manage stress levels.

2. Magnesium: Helps support relaxation, reduce stress, and improve sleep quality. Consider magnesium glycinate for better absorption.

3. Probiotics: Supports gut health, which is essential for overall hormonal balance. Look for broad-spectrum probiotics with at least 10 billion CFUs.

4. Fish Oil (Omega-3s): Supports brain health, reduces inflammation, and promotes heart health. Opt for high-quality, purified fish oil.

5. Vitamin C: A powerful antioxidant that helps reduce oxidative stress and supports the immune system.

6. Vitamin D: Essential for immune health and hormonal balance. Aim for a Vitamin D3 supplement if you are not getting enough sun exposure.

7. L-Theanine: Found in green tea, this amino acid promotes relaxation without sedation and supports mental clarity.

8. B-Complex: Essential for energy production and stress management, especially B5 and B6, which help reduce cortisol levels.

9. Melatonin: If you're having trouble with sleep, consider a low-dose melatonin supplement to improve your sleep quality and regulate circadian rhythms.

<u>Tools:</u>

1. Journaling for Stress Management: Keeping a daily journal can help reduce stress by allowing you to express emotions and reflect on your day.

2. A Quality Blender: To make your smoothies and detox drinks easier and more enjoyable, a powerful blender is a must-have for your kitchen.

3. Herbal Teas & Infusers: Stock up on calming teas like chamomile, peppermint, and lemon balm to unwind and relax throughout the day.

4. A Water Bottle with Hydration Reminders: Hydration is crucial during the detox process. A water bottle with hourly hydration reminders or a tracker can keep you on top of your water intake.

5. Foam Roller or Massage Tools: To reduce muscle tension and stress, regular use of a foam roller or handheld massager can help relieve built-up tension in your body.

6. Essential Oils & Diffusers: Lavender, eucalyptus, and peppermint essential oils can support relaxation, reduce stress, and help with sleep when used in a diffuser.

By utilizing this shopping list and supplementing with the right tools, you're well-equipped to support your cortisol detox journey with the right resources. Remember, the key is consistency and creating a supportive environment for your body to heal, balance, and thrive.

Printable Meal Planner Template

WEEKLY MEAL PLANNER

MONDAY ___/___/____

TUESDAY ___/___/____

WEDNESDAY___/___/____

THURSDAY ___/___/____

FRIDAY ___/___/____

SATURDAY ___/___/____

SUNDAY ___/___/____

SHOPPING LIST:

Conversion Chart

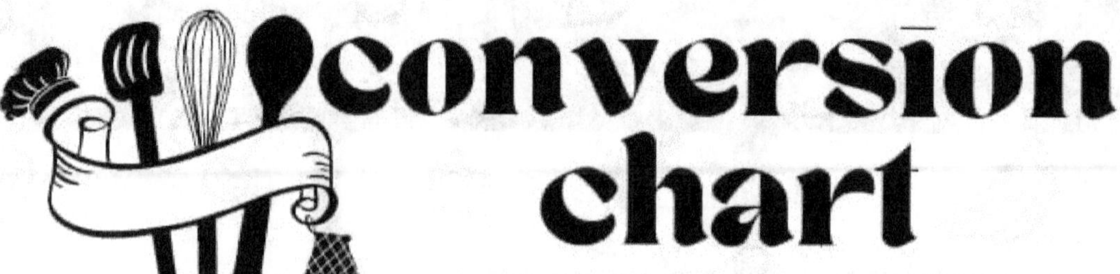

VOLUME MEASUREMENT CONVERSIONS

Cups	Tablespoons	Teaspoons	Milliliters
1/16 cup	1 tbsp	1 tsp	5ml
1/8 cup	2 tbsp	3 tsp	15 ml
1/4 cup	4 tbsp	6 tsp	30 ml
1/3 cup	5 1/3 tbsp	12 tsp	60 ml
1/2 cup	8 tbsp	16 tsp	80 ml
2/3 cup	10 2/3 tbsp	24 tsp	120 ml
3/4 cup	12 tbsp	32 tsp	160 ml
1 cup	16 tbsp	36 tsp	180 ml
		48 tsp	240 ml

1 QUART =
2 pints
4 cups
32 ounces
950 ml

1 PINT =
2 cups
16 ounces
480 ml

1 CUP =
16tbsp
8 ounces
240 ml

1/4 CUP =
4 tbsp
12 tsp
2 ounces
60 ml

1 TBSP =
3 tsp 1/2
ounce
15 ml

COOKING TEMPERATURE CONVERSIONS

Celcius/Centigrade $F=(C \times 1.8) + 32$

Fahrenheit $C=(F-32) \times 0.5556$

Ingredient Conversion

BAKING INGREDIENT CONVERSIONS

BUTTER

Cups	Grams
1/4 cup	57 grams
1/3 cup	76 grams
1/2 cup	113 grams
1 cup	227 grams

PACKED BROWN SUGAR

Cups	Grams	Ounces
1/4 cup	55 grams	1.9 oz
1/3 cup	73 grams	2.58 oz
1/2 cup	110 grams	3.88 oz
1 cup	220 grams	7.75 oz

ALL-PURPOSE FLOUR / CONFECTIONER'S SUGAR

Cups	Grams	Ounces
1/8 cup	16 grams	563 oz
1/4 cup	32 grams	1.13 oz
1/3 cup	43 grams	1.5 oz
1/2 cup	64 grams	2.25 oz
2/3 cup	85 grams	3 oz
3/4 cup	96 grams	3.38 oz
1 cup	128 grams	4.5 oz

GRANULATED SUGAR

Cups	Grams	Ounces
2 tbsp	25 grams	89 oz
1/4 cup	67 grams	1.78 oz
1/3 cup	50 grams	2.37 oz
1/2 cup	100 grams	3.55 oz
2/3 cup	134 grams	4.73 oz
3/4 cup	150 grams	5.3 oz
1 cup	201 grams	7.1 oz

9 798305 066456